The Advanced Practice Registered Nurse as a Prescriber

T0188311

The Advanced Practice Registered Nurse as a Prescriber

SECOND EDITION

Edited by

Louise Kaplan
Phd, ARNP, FNP-BC, FAANP, FAAN
Associate Professor
Washington State University
Vancouver, WA

Marie Annette Brown
Phd, ARNP, FNP-BC, FAANP, FAAN
Professor Emeritus
University of Washington
Seattle, WA

WILEY Blackwell

Registered Office(s)
John Wiley & Sons, Inc., 111 River Street, Hoboken, NJ 07030, USA
John Wiley & Sons Ltd, The Atrium, Southern Gate, Chichester, West Sussex, PO19 8SQ, UK

Editorial Office
9600 Garsington Road, Oxford, OX4 2DQ, UK

For details of our global editorial offices, customer services, and more information about Wiley products visit us at www.wiley.com.

Wiley also publishes its books in a variety of electronic formats and by print-on-demand. Some content that appears in standard print versions of this book may not be available in other formats.

Library of Congress Cataloging-in-Publication Data

Names: Kaplan, Louise, editor. | Brown, Marie Annette, editor.
Title: The advanced practice registered nurse as a prescriber / [edited by] Louise Kaplan, Marie Annette Brown.
Description: [Second edition]. | Hoboken, NJ : Wiley-Blackwell, 2021. | Preceded by The advanced practice registered nurse as a prescriber / Marie Annette Brown, Louise Kaplan. 2012. | Includes bibliographical references and index.
Identifiers: LCCN 2020039788 (print) | LCCN 2020039789 (ebook) | ISBN 9781119685579 (paperback) | ISBN 9781119685593 (adobe PDF) | ISBN 9781119685609 (epub)
Subjects: MESH: Advanced Practice Nursing–methods | Drug Prescriptions–nursing | Pharmaceutical Preparations–administration & dosage
Classification: LCC RT81.8(print) | LCC RT81.8(ebook) | NLM WY 128 | DDC 615.1/4–dc23
LC record available at https://lccn.loc.gov/2020039788
LC ebook record available at https://lccn.loc.gov/2020039789

Cover Design: Wiley
Cover Images: Nerthuz/getty Images

Set in 9/11 pt Palatino by SPi Global, Pondicherry, India

SKY680C48FD-5EE5-4AE5-8D4D-57E12012ABF9_030221

To my sons, Kai and Lee, for their understanding of the time I spent working on this project and advocating for advanced practice registered nurses. And to all the advanced practice registered nurses who have worked tirelessly to achieve full practice authority globally.

Louise Kaplan

To my husband, Eric Leberg, whose loving support and household management has sustained our family. To the patients, students, and colleagues who fueled my enthusiasm for a lifelong dedication to the advanced practice nursing role. And to my father, E. Moss Brown, who inspired me to believe that change is always possible and education is transformative.

Marie Annette Brown

Contents

Contributors

Editors
Louise Kaplan, PhD, ARNP, FNP-BC, FAANP, FAAN
Associate Professor
Washington State University
Vancouver, WA

Marie Annette Brown, PhD, ARNP, FNP-BC, FAANP, FAAN
Professor Emeritus
University of Washington
Seattle, WA

Contributors
Carolyn Dolan, JD, MSN, FNP-BC, PPCNP-BC
Professor
University of South Alabama
Mobile, AL

Pamela Stitzlein Davies, MS, ARNP, AGNP, RN-BC, FAANP
Nurse Practitioner
Adjunct Faculty, School of Health Sciences, Seattle Pacific University
Affiliate Instructor, School of Nursing, University of Washington
Seattle, WA

Tracy Klein, PhD, FNP, FAANP, FRE, FAAN
Associate Professor
Washington State University
Vancouver, WA

Donna L. Poole, MSN, ARNP, PMHCNS-BC
Nurse Practitioner
Peninsula Community Health Services
Poulsbo, WA

Preface

The purpose of this book is to provide advanced practice registered nurses (APRNs) with the information necessary to be fully informed, rational, and ethical prescribers. The genesis of this book was our teaching, practice, and research. Throughout our professional lives as nurse practitioners, we have experienced the demands, difficulties, and satisfaction inherent in accomplishing this goal.

In 2001, Washington State APRNs obtained prescriptive authority for Scheduled II–IV controlled substances. Our research revealed that when controlled substance prescribing was initially optional, many APRNs did not apply for this hard-won prescriptive authority. Some were reluctant to prescribe controlled substances. The slower-than-expected transition prompted our desire to develop a more in-depth understanding of how APRNs adopt the role of a prescriber. Likewise, our colleagues, the chapter authors, were inspired to share their prescribing wisdom gleaned from experience to mentor students and colleagues. They dedicated countless hours to the time-consuming and often difficult challenge of writing in addition to their ongoing professional demands.

We intend for this book to assist students who are adopting the role of APRN prescriber. We also intend to assist practicing APRNs who confront challenges as they transition to the full scope of the prescriber role. Most APRNs need to deepen their knowledge base as they fully implement new or expanded roles, particularly that of fully autonomous prescriber. Ultimately, this information will assist our colleagues across the nation and the world as they work to advance the profession to better serve patients. As APRNs enhance their prescribing expertise, they will enrich their professional opportunities to contribute to greater access and more patient-centered care. This expertise is also a basis on which we can create changes necessary to improve the quality of healthcare delivered to Americans.

Over the decades, multiple studies and national statements have supported the need for APRNs to practice to the full extent of their education and expertise. The major recommendation is that legal and regulatory barriers to APRN practice should be eliminated. We thank the APRNs who have worked tirelessly to do just that.

We acknowledge policymakers as well as local, state, and national nursing organizations that have been instrumental in advancing the profession of nursing. They honored the dream of advanced practice nursing pioneers who championed their creative innovation that is part of our professional heritage. We dedicate this book to the APRNs who continue the work needed to eliminate the barriers to full practice authority for all APRNs. We will not rest until we meet that goal!

Louise Kaplan and Marie Annette Brown

What Do APRN Prescribers Need to Understand?

1

Louise Kaplan and Marie Annette Brown

Today's healthcare transformations herald unprecedented opportunities for advanced practice registered nurses (APRNs) to provide and model patient-centered, evidence-based healthcare. As APRNs across the country increasingly secure full practice authority, they must seize the opportunity to become pace-setters for ethical, rational, and responsible prescribing. The vast majority of APRNs (nurse practitioners, nurse midwives, nurse anesthetists, and clinical nurse specialists) work with prescription medications on a daily basis. Many are unable to imagine a practice that does not include the ability to prescribe, provide, and/or manage medications for at least some of their patients. A goal of most APRNs, however, is utilization of a wide range of therapeutic modalities in the process of patient-centered care. This may include, but is not focused solely, on medications. Health promotion and disease prevention continue to be a hallmark of APRN practice.

At the same time, as the demand for prescriptive medications increases, prescriptive authority becomes an even more vital component of APRN practice. The number of prescriptions dispensed in 2018 was 5.8 billion, an increase of 2.7% from the prior year. During the same one-year period, opioid prescription use decreased by 17.1% (The IQVIA Institute, 2019). In order to appropriately meet the prescribing needs of patients, APRNs must have unencumbered, full prescriptive authority and practice.

Practice in today's complex, fast-paced healthcare delivery system in which there is a constant barrage of information can be overwhelming. Selection and monitoring of medication appropriate for patients is only one aspect of the complex process of prescribing. This book serves as an easily accessible reference to guide practicing APRNs through these challenges and supplements pharmacotherapeutic knowledge about specific medications. APRN students can also benefit from the content of this book. Standards for APRN programs specify a pharmacotherapeutic course as well as analysis of the APRN role (National Organization of Nurse Practitioner Faculties [NONPF], 2016). Educators must focus on teaching

The Advanced Practice Registered Nurse as a Prescriber, Second Edition. Edited by Louise Kaplan and Marie Annette Brown.
© 2021 John Wiley & Sons Ltd. Published 2021 by John Wiley & Sons Ltd.

the essential knowledge about pharmacokinetics, pharmacodynamics, and evidence-based drug treatment recommendations. Consequently, an in-depth discussion of the APRN's role as a prescriber is not usually found in the curriculum. The information included in this book has been compiled by experts to facilitate this discussion. The authors have used their clinical and professional experience to synthesize and organize key ideas on a wide variety of subjects. These include:

- What it means to be a prescriber
- The many facets of the prescriber role
- The legal, regulatory, and ethical responsibilities of APRNs who prescribe medications
- Who is a prescriber globally
- Managing difficult patient situations
- Strategies for assessing and addressing special considerations with controlled substances
- Authorizing medical marijuana

THE JOURNEY OF APRN PRESCRIPTIVE AUTHORITY

For decades, APRNs have invested innumerable hours in lobbying and regulatory work to advance APRN practice. They have solidified the APRN role, strengthened the foundation for APRN education, and expanded the knowledge base for expert practice. In the United States, APRNs in Idaho were the first authorized to prescribe medication in 1971, though it took six years for rules to be written and prescriptive authority to be implemented. Most, but not all, APRNs have now been granted prescriptive authority in all states. In California, for example, clinical nurse specialists and nurse anesthetists do not have prescriptive authority (Phillips, 2020). APRNs have repeatedly demonstrated that they provide effective, high-quality care, including prescribing medications. Nonetheless, APRNs in over half of the United States confront prescribing barriers imposed by state law on a daily basis. These barriers include requirements for supervision or collaboration, restrictions on prescribing controlled substances, and limitations on the type and quantity of medications that can be prescribed. Other barriers are imposed by federal law, such as the conditions under which an APRN may prescribe buprenorphine for substance use disorder.

As a consequence of prescribing barriers, many APRNs are unable to practice to the full extent of their educational preparation, knowledge, and abilities. This negatively affects patient care and the healthcare system overall. Practice constraints handicap the APRN who is unable to fulfill roles in outpatient and inpatient settings. These restrictions continue despite an increased demand for primary, specialty, and acute care providers, and the integration of primary care practices into large health systems. APRNs are in more demand with shortages of primary care providers, particularly to work with the underserved and as those living in rural areas increase. Nurses have a rich history of dedication to social justice and service to marginalized communities. Successful implementation of healthcare reforms in the years to come requires APRNs to be full partners with other health professionals, which necessitates the removal of barriers to allow APRNs to practice to the full extent of their education and expertise.

Washington State as an exemplar

A legislature must pass a bill to enable any changes in the scope of practice for ARPNs. The law typically cannot be implemented until the Board of Nursing adopts rules that specify the intent of the law. Scope of practice changes can take months to years to finalize. The history of APRN prescribing in Washington State begins with a 1977 law that authorized APRNs to prescribe legend drugs (medications requiring a prescription). However, dispensing medications and prescribing controlled substances were prohibited. The Board of Nursing then wrote rules that authorized APRNs to prescribe Schedule V drugs in 1982 and dispensing was added in 1983. It was not until 2000, after more than a decade of lobbying, that APRNs in Washington State obtained Schedule II–IV prescriptive authority.

This long-sought authority came with a price. For the first time since APRN practice was authorized by the legislature in 1973, physician involvement in APRN practice was mandated. APRNs who wanted II–IV prescriptive authority were required to obtain a Joint Practice Agreement (JPA) with a physician. Slowly over the next four years many APRNs began obtaining Schedule II–IV prescriptive authority. However, until the JPA was removed, over one-third of APRNs chose not to obtain II–IV prescriptive authority. This contradicted the expectation of APRN leaders in the state that nearly all APRNs would want the legal ability to prescribe controlled substances even if it was only utilized occasionally. We conducted research in Washington State to understand this unexpected phenomenon (Kaplan & Brown, 2004, 2007, 2009; Kaplan et al., 2006, 2010).

The findings of our research serve as a basis of understanding how APRNs may or may not transition to full prescriptive authority and practice when provided the opportunity. It also offers lessons learned about the need to prepare APRNs for a major transition in scope of practice. Change may cause concern for some who have adapted to the status quo, even if prescribing barriers limited their ability to practice. Many of these findings are discussed in Chapter 3. They will enhance your understanding about APRN prescribing practice, the consequences of limiting APRN practice, and the poorly understood experience of transition to a new scope of practice. It is not surprising, however, that APRNs respond to new practice authority with the natural ambivalence that accompanies most change processes.

OVERVIEW OF CHAPTERS

Chapter 2 guides the reader through an analysis of the role and responsibilities of the APRN as a prescriber. The ability to independently prescribe medications symbolizes the legitimacy of APRNs. The public often perceives the prescribing role as what defines the legitimacy of APRNs. This chapter includes an overview of the development of the APRN role and prescriptive authority, the essential nature of autonomy, and the process of transition to the prescribing role. The chapter emphasizes the shift from prescribing medication based on

3

professional preference and tradition to rational prescribing and evidence-based practice as strategies to achieve quality patient-centered care.

Given the multiple factors that influence the transition of the APRN to the prescriber role, there is an understandable degree of uncertainty and concern about prescribing. Challenges about the transition from a role that requires administration of medications and prescribed treatments as a registered nurse to the role of manager of care and prescriber as an APRN are delineated in Chapter 2. Change can be a professionally invigorating challenge rather than a distressing situation. It is understandable, however, that many role transitions are characterized by uncertainty and even fear along with the excitement and promise of change.

Chapter 3 highlights the multitude of challenges and opportunities that APRNs confront when prescribing medication. Laws, regulations, and policies, as well as the attitudes of other health professionals often limit prescribing. These are external barriers to an APRN's adoption of the prescribing role. Internal barriers also can diminish an APRN's interest in fully autonomous practice and can be overlooked in an analysis of barriers to APRN prescribing. Internal barriers to "stepping up" are invisible or unacknowledged factors within the individual APRN, and include personal characteristics such as conflict avoidance or the "need to be liked." Strategies to overcome internal and external prescribing barriers are offered as a way to generate enthusiasm among APRNs for facilitating change as well as to deepen their courage to take the inherent risks in full practice authority.

Chapter 4 details the laws, regulations, and professional issues that affect prescribing. These include state laws, Board of Nursing rules, and interprofessional constraints. Fully autonomous prescribing is contrasted with examples of restricted prescribing authority. Restrictions include the requirement for physician supervision, the need to use formularies, and the lack of authority to prescribe controlled substances.

The *Consensus Model for APRN Regulation, Licensure, Accreditation, Certification and Education* was a landmark agreement developed over several years of dialogue and negotiation by representatives of education, state Boards of Nursing, and professional practice organizations. Discussion of the Consensus Model highlights the need for standardized regulation that achieves fully autonomous practice with full prescriptive authority and universal adoption of the term APRN. This chapter can assist APRNs across the nation to visualize and positively anticipate their future practice and prescribing.

Chapter 5 provides an overview of APRN and registered nurse (RN) prescribing globally. Overall, more countries have adopted RN prescribing than APRN prescribing. The nurse practitioner (NP) role is the most widespread of the four APRN roles, particularly because midwifery is not always a nursing role worldwide. The chapter discusses different approaches to RN and NP prescribing such as through task sharing, formularies, and independent authority.

Chapter 6 coaches APRNs to deal with difficult and often complex clinical situations that are inherent in human relationships and professional interactions, even among experienced and dedicated APRNs. These situations often create anxiety and may even generate anger when the APRN feels ill-prepared to deal with them. The basic tenet is that these are not *problem patients* but situations for which the APRN needs more knowledge, skill, and insight from self-reflection. Examples of these situations include dealing with patients who are or appear to be seeking controlled substances, are angry, request inappropriate care such as antibiotics for a viral infection, and who violate boundaries. One goal of the discussion is to enhance understanding of why these difficult situations develop and how they can impact patient-centered care. Specific strategies to identify difficult situations, respond to them appropriately, and build competence as a supportive and courageous APRN prescriber are discussed.

Chapter 7 discusses the characteristic clinical challenges inherent in prescribing controlled substances and the strategies to address them. This information is particularly relevant in the midst of an opioid epidemic in the United States. Accurate definitions of terms related to drug use or misuse and their application provide a rationale to create more skillful communication with patients around complex and sensitive issues. The use of deliberate, concrete approaches to prescribing controlled substances such as an opioid use agreement with a patient are key strategies to build prescribing expertise. A wide range of topics is discussed and include: "universal precautions" for use with the prescription of controlled substances; the assessment, management, and monitoring of patients with chronic non-cancer pain; clinical guidelines; the use of prescription drug monitoring programs; providing medication therapy for people with substance use disorder; and standards for the identification of a patient who misuses substances.

Chapter 8 helps APRNs become savvy prescribers and avoid missteps during their career. A series of case exemplars highlight common mistakes that resulted in legal action. Prescriptive authority for APRNs is based on federal laws about controlled substances, state laws, and the standard of care necessary across various classes of drugs. These exemplars highlight the role of Boards of Nursing, malpractice attorneys when a lawsuit is filed, the Drug Enforcement Administration, and government auditors who monitor nursing facilities. An overview of malpractice insurance and risk mitigation provides the APRN with strategies to protect one's practice and prescribe safely.

Chapter 9 introduces the rapidly evolving landscape of medical marijuana which is now legal in several countries worldwide. Although illegal at the federal level in the United States, over three-dozen states and jurisdictions have legal medical, and in some instances recreational, marijuana. While APRNs do not "prescribe" medical marijuana, in some of the states one or more of the APRN roles may provide patients with "authorizations" to use medical marijuana. This chapter includes a brief overview of marijuana as a drug, federal and state law, the typical process to provide an authorization, standards of care, and the evidence-base for medical marijuana. While no APRN is required to provide an authorization in states where it is permitted, all APRNs will want to know the law in their state of practice and be prepared to answer questions and use an evidence-based approach to assist patients in their decision making.

CONCLUSION
Ultimately, this book is more than a guide and reference for building and enhancing prescribing expertise. It honors the work of APRNs who use

prescriptive authority to provide comprehensive quality care. The book is a tribute to the countless number of APRNs who have worked tirelessly for full practice and prescriptive authority and those who have invested decades of their careers to become expert prescribers. Toward that end, we hope the book is an inspiration to students. You are the next generation of APRNs who are urgently needed to join current advocates in the efforts to obtain full prescriptive authority nationwide. We look forward to the day this is achieved.

REFERENCES

Kaplan, L., & Brown, M.A. (2004). Prescriptive authority and barriers to NP practice. *Nurse Practitioner, 29*(3), 28–35.

Kaplan, L., & Brown, M.A. (2007). The transition of nurse practitioners to changes in prescriptive authority. *Journal of Nursing Scholarship, 39*(2), 184–190.

Kaplan, L., & Brown, M.A. (2009). Prescribing controlled substances: Perceptions, realities and experiences in Washington State. *American Journal for Nurse Practitioners, 12*(3), 44–51, 53.

Kaplan, L., Brown, M.A., Andrilla, H., & Hart, L.G. (2006). Barriers to autonomous practice. *The Nurse Practitioner, 31*(1), 57–63.

Kaplan, L., Brown, M.A., & Donohue, J.S. (2010). Prescribing controlled substances: How NPs in Washington are making a difference. *The Nurse Practitioner, 35*(5), 47–53.

National Organization of Nurse Practitioner Faculties. (2016). Criteria for evaluation of nurse practitioner programs. Retrieved from https://cdn.ymaws.com/www.nonpf.org/resource/resmgr/docs/evalcriteria2016final.pdf. (Accessed 7 September 2020.)

Phillips, S.J. (2020). 32nd annual APRN legislative update: Improving access to high-quality, safe and effective healthcare. *The Nurse Practitioner, 45*(1), 28–55.

The IQVIA Institute. (2019). Medicine use and spending in the U.S. Retrieved from https://www.iqvia.com/insights/the-iqvia-institute/reports/medicine-use-and-spending-in-the-us-a-review-of-2018-and-outlook-to-2023. (Accessed 7 September 2020.)

Embracing the Prescriber Role as an APRN

2

Louise Kaplan and Marie Annette Brown

This chapter emphasizes the importance of prescriptive authority as a component of advanced practice registered nurse (APRN) practice. An overview describes the development of, and transition to, the APRN role, with an emphasis on prescribing. The framework for rational prescribing rests on knowledge of the patient, knowledge about the nature of the health problem, and treatment using evidence-based guidelines, standards of care, and strategies for promoting appropriate medication use.

The ability to independently prescribe medications is a hallmark symbol of the legitimacy of advanced practice registered nurses (Aprns). The public often perceives the prescriber role as what 'defines' an APRN. Therefore, a goal of APRNs is full practice authority and professional integrity to provide comprehensive patient care. APRNs prescribe medications not only to meet the needs of individual patients and families but also to meet societal needs and the expectations of a fully autonomous profession like nursing. Prescribing is a component of each of the four APRN roles: certified registered nurse anesthetist (CRNA), certified nurse-midwife (CNM), clinical nurse specialist (CNS), and nurse practitioner (NP). Prescribing is within the scope of practice for NPs and CNMs in all 50 US states but is more limited for CNSs and CRNAs (National Council of State Boards of Nursing [NCSBN], 2020). This chapter provides information for APRNs to enhance expertise and confidence for successful adoption of the fully autonomous prescriber role.

DEVELOPMENT OF THE APRN ROLE

The APRN role began with nurse anesthetists in the late 1800s, preceding anesthesiologists by several decades. Nurse midwives became established in the United States in the early 1900s, while the CNS role evolved in the 1940s and 1950s (Dunphy, 2018). The NP role, formally developed in 1965, has grown the most rapidly, with NPs becoming the largest group of APRNs. Legislatures enacted laws that provided a scope of practice for APRNs consistent with their educational preparation. Over time, APRNs have established themselves as

---

The Advanced Practice Registered Nurse as a Prescriber, Second Edition. Edited by Louise Kaplan and Marie Annette Brown.
© 2021 John Wiley & Sons Ltd. Published 2021 by John Wiley & Sons Ltd.

members of the healthcare workforce with a distinct role, a unique education, and essential knowledge and skills to provide care.

APRN scope of practice varies across the United States according to state laws that are the basis of regulation. Advanced practice nursing is controlled by licensure, accreditation, credentialing, and educational preparation, and practice opportunities which require greater expertise. Variation in APRN roles also results from organizational policies that may support or constrain practice. APRNs are responsible for maintaining a high ethical standard in practice, generating knowledge, and appraising and translating evidence to provide quality, comprehensive, patient-centered care.

Although there has been significant progress in the utilization of APRNs, constraints on consumers' access to APRNs, legal limitations, and absence of full practice authority in all states continue to limit APRN practice. Constraints on APRNs that limit their practice are most likely due to concerns about professional competition because extensive data exist about APRN quality of care. For decades, studies have demonstrated that APRN care is as or more effective than care delivered by physicians (Brown & Grimes, 1995; Congressional Budget Office, 1979; DesRoches et al., 2017; Dulisse & Cromwell, 2010; Horrocks et al., 2002; Jennings et al., 2015; Landsperger et al., 2016; Laurant et al., 2018; Lenz et al., 2004; Newhouse et al., 2011; Ohman-Strickland et al., 2008; Prescott & Driscoll, 1980; Safriet, 1992; Simonson et al., 2007; Spitzer et al., 1974; Wright et al., 2011). Many of these studies also validated widespread acceptance of the APRN role and high satisfaction with APRN care.

Increasing demands for APRNs and assessment of their cost-effectiveness are powerful factors expected to influence the eventual removal of legal barriers remaining in many states. Concurrently, an improved regulatory environment, especially in relationship to prescriptive authority, has helped legitimize and distinguish the APRN role. In states where NPs have full practice authority which includes complete prescriptive authority, the difference between NPs and physician assistants (PAs) is more apparent and often provides an increased incentive to hire NPs. PA practice, which includes prescribing, is always supervised by and is legally linked with a physician. Furthermore, implementation of the *Consensus Model for APRN Regulation, Licensure, Accreditation, Certification and Education* (see Chapter 4) can assist APRNs to attain full practice authority.

Autonomy is an important professional concept related to full practice authority. The nursing literature on advanced practice confirms it has been difficult to achieve (Ulrich & Soeken, 2005; Weiland, 2008), mainly due to resistance from organized medicine. Even in the presence of team-based healthcare, some physicians perceive themselves as the apparent leader or supervisor, which reflects a desire to limit and/or control APRN practice for multiple reasons. Physician control of APRN prescribing often has financial benefits for the physician who is paid for "supervision" that is unnecessary given the educational preparation of APRNs in pharmacotherapeutic content. Physician control of nursing practice is inconsistent with true APRN professional autonomy. Autonomy is also a professional and personal sense of the unfettered ability to make decisions in practice when legally granted to a professional through the endorsement of society. *"Having genuine NP practice"* emerged as the major theme of a qualitative study about NP autonomy that was expressed in four major subthemes: relationships, self-reliance, self-empowerment, and defending the NP role (Weiland, 2015). This involved the meaning of the NPs' practice experience and experience of being an NP. Autonomy extends beyond legal authority. "It is not just in action but in thought that we create our autonomy" (Kaplan & Brown, 2006, p. 37).

DEVELOPMENT OF THE APRN ROLE AND PRESCRIPTIVE AUTHORITY
Prescriptive authority
Prescriptive authority is the legal ability to prescribe drugs and devices, a practice regulated by the states. One aspect of prescriptive authority, controlled substances (CSs), is specifically regulated by the federal government through the Drug Enforcement Administration (DEA) which enforces the Controlled Substances Act of 1970 (Title 21 – Food and Drugs, 1993). Some states have additional regulations and requirements related to prescribing CSs.

Obtaining prescriptive authority for APRNs has presented significant challenges nationwide. Even when prescriptive authority is supported in new legislation, significant roadblocks to implementation often occur, particularly those placed by physicians. In 1971, for example, Idaho became the first state to pass legislation that recognized the NP role and granted prescriptive authority. Although the first Idaho NP entered practice in 1972, opposition from the Board of Medicine resulted in more than one-dozen drafts of the prescriptive authority rules. The rules were not adopted until 1977, making Idaho the first state to implement prescriptive authority for NPs (personal communication, S. Evans, December 28, 2009). Nearly 30 years later, in 2006, Georgia became the last state to pass a law granting APRNs authority to "order" medications, a variant of prescribing (Phillips, 2007). An example of a current barrier exists in Colorado. After program completion, an APRN must first qualify for provisional prescriptive authority (RXN-P). Within three years of receiving RXN-P status, the APRN must complete a 1000 hour mentorship with a physician or APRN with full prescriptive authority (RXN) and develop an articulated plan for safe prescribing to receive full prescriptive authority (Code of Colorado Regulation, 2017).

ADAPTING TO THE APRN'S ROLE AS PRESCRIBER
Transition to the prescribing role
One of the greatest responsibilities for an APRN is that of prescription medication management. Prescribing is not typically a part of the registered nurse (RN) role in most countries including the US, and often requires a major paradigm shift to transition from administering drugs to selecting and prescribing medications. Consequently, the individual APRN's transition to the prescriber role involves a union between knowledge of pharmacotherapeutics and socialization to the role. APRNs begin gaining knowledge and competencies throughout their graduate education and continue this process through practice. Role socialization to become a prescriber is initiated during APRN education and likewise is part of continuing professional development.

Transition to the prescriber role is part of the larger role transition that the APRN experiences first as a student, then as a novice practitioner, and when scope of practice changes. Schumacher and Meleis (1994) identified five factors that influence role transition. These continue to be relevant for APRNs in today's practice arena. They are:

1. Personal meaning of the transition
2. Degree of planning for the transition
3. Environmental barriers and supports
4. Level of knowledge and skill
5. Expectations.

Identification of these factors may allow the APRN to prepare ways for a smooth transition, although there are other dimensions of transition that also need to be considered.

Students in APRN programs typically experience a role transition process that involves role confusion and role strain, including tension, frustration, and anxiety (Brykcznski, 2019). Role acquisition extends to the practicing APRN. The first year of practice is an especially challenging one. A study by Brown and Olshansky (1998) identified four stages in the transition to the primary care NP role. These are laying the foundation, launching, meeting the challenge, and broadening the perspective. Table 2.1 describes these stages. The study findings revealed the importance of skillful mentors who serve as a compass to guide the NP and serve as a source of information and support. Access to a mentor can be especially important in respect to adoption of the role of a prescriber, which brings a special set of challenges.

Table 2.1 Nurse practitioners' experience during the first year of primary care practice

Stage 1: Laying the Foundation

    Recuperating from school
    Negotiating the bureaucracy
    Looking for a job
    Worrying

Stage 2: Launching

    Feeling real
    Getting through the day
    Battling time
    Confronting anxiety

Stage 3: Meeting the challenge

    Increasing competence
    Gaining confidence
    Acknowledging system problems

Stage 4: Broadening the perspective

    Developing system savvy
    Affirming oneself
    Upping the ante

Source: From Brown and Olshansky (1998), reprinted with permission from Wolters Kluwer Health.

Grappling with general questions about prescribing contributes to professional development and strengthens prescribing expertise during an APRN's career.

• What is the APRN's role in a particular healthcare setting?
• What is the APRN's relationship to a collaborating or supervising physician when this relationship is required by state law?
• What if I disagree with a physician about the choice of the most appropriate medication?
• How does one adapt when relocating to a state with a different scope of practice?

General questions are often followed by more specific patient-centered questions. For example:

• Am I making the right medication choice?
• Is medication the most appropriate treatment option or should non-pharmacologic approaches be used at this point in the treatment trajectory?
• What type of antibiotic should be prescribed to treat a methicillin-resistant *Staphylococcus aureus* infection?
• When should a person with type 2 diabetes consider beginning insulin therapy?
• What is the appropriate medication to manage acute, subacute, or chronic pain?

When faced with the reality of determining specific practice decisions, particularly those about prescribing, the novice APRN may experience a sense of uncertainty. Novice APRNs enter advanced practice step-by-step, decision-by-decision. Experience is a remarkable teacher, and, gradually, APRNs develop their professional practice and role identity which includes competence in prescribing. APRNs need time to transition into their new role. It is key, however, to emphasize that a novice APRN receiving the wisdom of a trusted colleague is different than the "requirement" for physician supervision. All novice prescribers, including physicians, benefit from this type of support.

Another aspect of adopting the APRN role is to contend with constraints imposed on all prescribers by health plans and healthcare delivery systems. For example, insurers promote the use of generic medications by requiring higher co-payments or refusing to pay for some brand-name drugs. Healthcare systems such as the Veterans Health Administration (VA) and health maintenance organizations such as Kaiser Permanente increasingly use formularies. These limit the medications that are paid for by the health plan, which promotes the use of generic drugs. For the most part, use of generic drugs is an important approach to address skyrocketing US healthcare costs, especially if they produce the same outcomes as branded medication. There are situations, however, in which the patient responds differently to generic vs. branded drugs. The APRN can be limited to only the generic, which compromises patient care. When a branded or non-covered medication is necessary, a particularly time-consuming, infuriating, and complex challenge is the prior authorization process. Providers must obtain permission from the health plan to make an exception to the policy (Jones et al., 2019).

In the practice setting, the APRN may be confronted with challenges to adopting the role of prescriber. In states with considerable limitations on autonomous prescribing, restrictions may be stipulated in practice agreements. Furthermore, specific clinical practice settings or individual characteristics of the collaborating physicians may limit the APRNs' decision making, especially when an APRN choses a medication that differs from his or her preference. Collaborative practice agreements may specify that the physician has the ability to override an APRN's prescribing decision.

The shift from professional preference and tradition to evidence-based practice has been shown to be a key strategy for achieving quality patient care. Improved models for prescribing that increase the effectiveness of care and reduce error and cost are emerging from the rational prescribing and evidence-based care movements. These models use clinical practice guidelines and electronic health records, exert more control over pharmaceutical marketing, and promote standards for formularies.

Commitment to these evidence-informed models is essential for APRNs to improve quality and safety. Recently educated APRNs, steeped in careful attention to rational and evidence-based prescribing, are likely to encounter situations with colleagues who may be unaware of current medication information. These situations often require assertiveness and communication skills that facilitate collegial sharing about continuously changing knowledge.

Prescriptive authority and responsibility

Changes to prescriptive authority for APRNs may be sponsored by legislators with limited understanding of the clinical abilities of the APRN (Safriet, 2002). Prescriptive authority carries responsibilities, even in states where collaboration or supervision is required. APRNs are accountable to patients, colleagues, the nursing profession, and society for their actions, decisions, and practice. As with any aspect of practice, errors or negligence in prescribing may result in disciplinary or legal action.

With all of the factors that influence the transition of the APRN as a prescriber, there will be a degree of uncertainty, and often anxiety, about prescribing. The transition from the RN role as the medication administrator to the APRN role as the medication prescriber can be viewed as a professionally invigorating challenge or as a distressing situation.

Professional relationships

Implementation of the APRN role requires the development of strong relationships with other healthcare professionals, patients, the profession, and society. The time and effort needed to establish and maintain these relationships may be demanding. The transition from the RN to the APRN role may change APRNs' relationships with patients less than it changes relationships with other healthcare professionals. The most dramatic change for APRNs is likely to occur with physicians. APRNs' level of prescribing expertise and the legal requirements of the prescriptive authority will influence relationships with physicians. A physician may be a colleague in the true sense of the word or may serve as a consultant or supervisor. The relationship between an APRN and a physician at its best will be similar to one's relationship with another APRN colleague: fulfilling, supportive, and truly collaborative with the interests of the patient at its core. A problematic relationship with a collaborating or supervising physician can serve as a barrier to APRN practice and compromise patient care. In those situations, APRNs may experience isolation, invalidation, and marginalization.

It is essential for APRNs to enhance their skills to manage and improve contentious professional relationships. APRNs who skillfully challenge and improve strained collegial relationships can build professional acceptance for all APRNs as well as enhance the quality of their own work life. These are situations where support and collaboration from other APRNs may be particularly effective. Some practices, however, may employ only one APRN, and time for collegial interaction at one's workplace may be limited.

The practice relationships that are legally required between APRNs and physicians vary from state to state. The majority of states still require some type of collaborative practice and some limit prescribing for specific medications or controlled drugs. For example, Alabama has one of the most restrictive scopes of advanced practice in the United States. Neither CNSs nor CRNAs may prescribe. For NPs and CNMs, prescribing limits include the following:

- The drug type, dosage, quantity prescribed, and number of refills shall be authorized and signed by the collaborating physician.
- The drug shall be on the formulary recommended by the joint committee and adopted by the State Board of Medical Examiners and the Board of Nursing.
- A certified registered NP or a CNM may not initiate a call-in prescription in the name of the collaborating physician for any drug, whether legend or CS, which the certified registered NP is not authorized to prescribe under the protocol, with certain exceptions (Alabama State Board of Nursing, 2020).

In states with restrictive practice laws, APRNs may be subject to direct oversight of a physician regardless of their expertise. Beyond a legal requirement for collaboration or supervision, physicians may view APRNs differently from how APRNs view themselves. A study in a midwestern VA region investigated NPs' and physicians' perceptions of the NP role, the degree of collegiality between the NPs and physicians, and the extent to which NPs felt accepted (Fletcher et al., 2007). NPs viewed themselves as autonomous and utilized physician collaborators in a consultation role. Physicians viewed the NPs as "extenders" (who serve a purpose for the MDs) to "free-up their time." In both groups, the relationship between the physician and NP was seen as collegial, and physicians were satisfied with NP practice contributions. These data highlight how, despite interprofessional relationships that seem collegial and satisfying to both APRNs and MDs, physicians may maintain a traditional, hierarchical view of APRNs promoted by organized medicine. At the same time, there are many clinical settings where APRNs are viewed as colleagues. One study of primary care physicians and NPs in Missouri, a restricted practice state, revealed how physicians and NPs had similar views on many issues and their responses to each other lacked defensiveness or conflict. Moreover, NPs did not view physicians as impediments to their work with patients and physicians respected NPs and viewed their skills favorably (Kraus & DuBois, 2017).

Relationships with pharmacists are particularly important for the APRN prescriber. The pharmacist is the expert on pharmacological agents, while the APRN applies knowledge of medications contextually to the patient situation, patient preferences, and expectations of best practice. Ideally, APRNs work with pharmacists as colleagues who have the same goal of appropriate and safe medication management and a commitment to quality patient care.

A patient's pharmacological management may involve collaboration with a specialized practitioner, for example, a physician or APRN who practices in endocrinology. Different collaborative approaches may be used.

- A patient consultation is made with the specialist for evaluation and development of a medication regimen. The regimen is implemented and monitored by the APRN.
- A patient is referred to a specialist who assumes care for specific health needs of the patient. The APRN typically maintains the role as the coordinator of care.

It is essential, however, that patients with a variety of complex problems who receive care from multiple specialists who prescribe medications have coordinated care and medications monitored by the primary care APRN.

Strategies for success as a prescriber

Changes in evidence-based practice, patient-centered outcomes research, and the introduction of new medications require regular review of patient medication regimens. A professional development plan will help the APRN utilize the most current evidence in medication management.

Participation in lifelong learning is the essence of a professional development plan. Different forms of lifelong learning may include collegial mentoring by another APRN, participation in professional organizations, informal networking with colleagues, peer review, and continuing education seminars or online training that focuses on current medication management approaches. Forty states require demonstration of continued competency to maintain licensure/recognition as an APRN; requirements vary from continuing education beyond the RN license requirement, pharmacology education, maintenance of national certification, practice, and peer review (NCSBN, 2020).

Efficient time management hinges on the APRN's medication management expertise. One approach to enhance prescribing effectiveness is to develop a "personal formulary" of medications one typically prescribes from different drug classes or for specific health conditions. This personal formulary is developed through current evidence, experience, patient feedback and responses to medications, and financial considerations.

Besides the use of a personal formulary, the APRN may employ strategies for prescribing drugs that save time and reduce the incidence of errors in medication management. Electronic prescribing reduces errors associated with illegibly written and improper prescriptions which often require a pharmacist to seek clarification. Nonetheless, errors related to electronic prescribing occur within hospital and community settings from both the provider side and the pharmacist side (Abramson, 2015; Alex et al., 2016). The need to communicate with pharmacists continues and will facilitate medication monitoring and prescription renewal.

In the interest of safety, it is recommended that patients use one pharmacy only. In situations when the APRN is concerned a patient is misusing medications, there are programs through private and public health plans that can mandate use of one pharmacy only. Use of one pharmacy reduces medication errors, drug interactions, and multiple prescriptions from multiple providers for the same medication, particularly scheduled drugs. An example of a public program that can mandate one pharmacy only is the Washington State Medicaid program known as *Patient Review and Coordination* which addresses overall excess utilization of services including medication use. Clients assigned to the program have had a 33% decrease in emergency room use, 37% decrease in office visits, and 24% decrease in prescriptions (Washington State Health Care Authority, 2020).

Novice prescribers may require an extensive amount of time to consult references, electronic medication guides, and clinical guidelines to select the most appropriate medication and write prescriptions. Electronic health records (EHRs) usually provide medication choices written with the generic rather than the brand name. Sometimes the desired dose or delivery approach is not specified in the dropdown menu, so consultation with peers can be especially useful in adapting to a new EHR. Because the development of expertise will take time and occurs over months and years, APRNs are encouraged to have realistic expectations of the time required to develop competence and be patient with themselves during this process.

An analysis of how patients, prescribers, experts, and patient advocates view the prescription choice process identified five important factors: information, relationship, patient variation, practitioner variation, and role expectations. The researchers noted that "decisions regarding the selection and use of prescription medications are made by multiple individuals, at multiple times, in multiple locations, under different contexts and viewpoints. The prescription choice process may be complicated further by various abilities, beliefs, and motivations held by those involved in the decisions" (Schommer et al., 2009, p. 167). Indeed, prescribing medications may appear easy but in actuality is complex.

BARRIERS TO TRANSITIONING TO THE PRESCRIBER ROLE

Some barriers may impede rather than facilitate role transition and the APRN's assumption of the prescriber role. Prescribing is the aspect of the APRN role most commonly constrained by legal requirements for physician collaboration or supervision. Prior to obtaining CS prescriptive authority, Washington State

APRNs experienced numerous barriers to assure their patients received the CSs they needed. The three most common barriers were physician concern about possible liability as a collaborator, a physician and NP choosing different drugs, and physician reluctance to prescribe drugs selected by the NP (Kaplan & Brown, 2004). For APRNs in states with required collaborative agreements or supervision for prescribing, thoughtful conversations with a physician colleague may reduce misconceptions and discord. Even in states with full practice authority, physicians who employ APRNs may expect to have input into an APRN's prescribing decisions.

A FRAMEWORK FOR PRESCRIBING
Rational prescribing
Rational prescribing rests on knowledge of the patient, knowledge about the nature of the health problem, and treatment using evidence-based guidelines, standards of care, strategies for promoting medication use, health plan coverage, and socioeconomic factors. With this information, the APRN and the patient make a shared decision through consideration of the benefits and burdens in the patient's particular situation. Both need to be mindful of the APRN's responsibility to act in the best interest of the patient. There are four general elements to rational prescribing: knowledge of the patient, knowledge of the disease and standard management, patient education and shared decision making, and maintaining a trust relationship with the patient.

Knowledge of the patient
Proper prescribing of medications requires careful evaluation of the patient with consideration of the patient's health history, medication history, and physical assessment. A complete medication history includes herbal and non-prescription medications, prescription medications, recreational drugs, and all drug reactions. This more comprehensive approach involves assessing allergic responses, drug interactions, and family genetic propensities. Thirty-three states, the District of Columbia, Guam, Puerto Rico, and the US Virgin Islands have legalized medical marijuana and 14 states and territories have approved adult use marijuana (National Conference of State Legislatures, 2020). It is important to know about patient use of marijuana to be able to effectively guide patients with evidence-based information when the APRN is authorized by law (see Chapter 9).

One important but often forgotten area of assessment is the patient's ability to manage his or her own medications. Names of drugs and the purpose of each drug may pose challenges for many patients. Assessment of the patient's motivation, cognitive abilities, attitudes about medication management, self-care, readiness to learn, health literacy, occupation, and educational background is essential to avoid false assumptions about the patient's ability to follow the healthcare plan. For example, a provider may incorrectly assume that a patient who is a nurse does not require the same counseling as other patients about medication side effects. Some patients with unusual chronic problems may be more knowledgeable about their illness and medication management than the APRN. Others may be inexperienced, misinformed, and/or uninformed about the medications they use.

Knowledge of the disease and standard management

APRNs continually gain experience and knowledge of the constantly changing area of pharmacological treatment. Rational prescribing is a method of drug management that is well established in international health and has become a cornerstone for prescribing medications to avoid adverse drug events (ADEs). The World Health Organization (2002) defined the rational use of medicines as follows:

> Patients receive medications appropriate to their clinical needs, in doses that meet their own individual requirements for an adequate period of time, and the lowest cost to them and their community.

The risk factors for ADEs are patient-related, drug-specific, and clinician-specific. Older adults and children are both more vulnerable to an ADE; however, polypharmacy, the strongest risk factor for an ADE, is more common in adults. Four types of medications – antidiabetic drugs, oral anticoagulants, antiplatelet agents, and opioid pain medication – account for more than 50% of emergency department visits for ADEs in Medicare patients (Agency for Healthcare Research and Quality, 2020).

Some medications may not be appropriate for specific populations. The Beers Criteria and Screening Tool of Older Persons' Potentially Inappropriate Prescriptions (STOPP) can be used in a complementary manner to evaluate potentially inappropriate medications for adults 65 years or older (Blanco-Reina et al., 2014). The Beers Criteria identify medications that should be avoided because they are ineffective, they pose an unnecessarily high risk, or there is a safer alternative. The criteria also identify medications that should not be prescribed when the person has specific health problems. The STOPP criteria are organized according to physiological systems and overcome some of the limitations of the Beers Criteria.

Rational prescribing also involves prescription drug costs. One way to reduce costs without compromising high-quality care is the use of generic drugs. Brand-name drugs are usually prescribed for patients who have a strong preference or when generics fail or are not available. Safety of brand-name drugs can also be an issue particularly when a medication is new to the market. There is less information about potential adverse consequences that may become apparent only after years of widespread use. Box 2.1 presents some strategies for improving rational prescribing.

Many professional organizations publish clinical guidelines and standards of care that include strategies for prescribing. All APRNs, especially novice practitioners, can benefit from these and other resources. A key aspect of rational prescribing is documentation of decisions. Refer to Chapter 8 for a full discussion on the importance of documentation.

Patient education and shared decision making

One of the greatest strengths of APRNs is the ability to develop a therapeutic relationship with patients and provide education. APRNs also facilitate patient learning about pharmacological and non-pharmacological options. Shared decision making with the patient will result in an individualized plan of care

---

Box 2.1 Strategies for improving rational prescribing

- Resist prescribing for minor, self-limiting, or non-specific symptoms.
- Avoid influences that can cloud rational decision making.
- Do not accept gifts that even have the *appearance* of affecting your decision making.
- Balance information received from the pharmaceutical industry with objective, unbiased sources.
- Encourage patients to seek out non-biased sources of information.
- Use evidence-based guidelines and electronic or current print references to assist in prescribing.
- Review patient medications during each visit.
- Emphasize lifestyle changes and always teach non-pharmacological management.
- Simplify and discontinue medications whenever possible.
- Avoid empirical treatment.
- Reduce the number of pharmacies and providers whenever possible.
- Titrate medication slowly.
- Monitor non-prescription drugs and treatments.

Sources: Farrell et al., 2003; Fick et al., 2003; Fulton & Allen, 2005; McVeigh, 2001.

---

that the patient is more likely to adopt. Emphasis on "knowing the patient" and exploring their attitudes about medication use helps practitioners avoid prescribing when the patient has no intention of taking a medication. A powerful but often overlooked question is imperative: *How do YOU feel about the idea of taking this medication?*

Only the United States and New Zealand have direct-to-consumer advertisement about medications with both positive and negative effects on patients (Filipova, 2019). Advertisements inform people about medications and symptoms related to certain disorders, promote information seeking, increase use of appropriate drugs when underuse is present, and improve the patient's perception of their interactions with providers. Advertisements may also influence consumers to request unnecessary or inappropriate medications or interfere with medication adherence, all of which makes rational prescribing more difficult (DeFrank et al., 2019). APRNs, through education and counseling, can help patients understand these external influences and make an appropriate decision that reflects rational treatment choices.

Shared decision making should include a discussion of whether the use of medication is physically and financially sustainable, the accessibility of the treatment, and the ease of use. Patients should be informed of the most common and serious side effects as well as key monitoring tests that contribute to patient safety. For example, a psychiatric NP will need to monitor levels of lithium at periodic levels to avoid toxicity. Many patients have conducted considerable Internet research prior to their visit which prompts medication questions or issues. Through education, a patient is provided with relevant facts to make a decision about whether to take a medication. Consent is typically verbal, but there may be situations in which written consent is obtained such as when prescribing a medication "off label," i.e. when a medication is prescribed for a reason not approved by the Food and Drug Administration (FDA).

The APRN should work collaboratively with pharmacists who are experts in their field to educate patients about their medications. Patients may read information about medications and become fearful of the potential side effects and thus do not fill the prescription or do not take the medicine once obtained from the pharmacy. This requires a balance between providing too much and providing too little information about medications. At a minimum, patients should be sufficiently informed to understand the action of a drug, the dosage, and the most common and severe adverse reactions. They also need to be informed about how to handle common problems, missing a dose, follow-up if the drug is not effective, and under what conditions the medication can be discontinued.

It is also important to provide guidance about how long the patient should expect to take the medication, particularly for non-communicable conditions. A guiding principle of prescribing is to use the lowest dose for the shortest period of time possible. An ideal medication is one that is effective with minimal or no side effects and is low cost. Sometimes the patient's health issue resolves. Lifestyle modifications such as exercise and sodium reduction may result in lowered blood pressure. In other instances a person may need antihypertensive medication despite these modifications.

Maintaining a trust relationship with the patient

APRN prescribing is based on recommendations about medications that reflect the patient's best interests. Decisions also reflect patient preferences. Additionally, the APRN should guard against participating in relationships that conflict with the patient's best interests. Licensed prescribers in the District of Columbia's Medicare Part D program who accepted gifts from pharmaceutical companies were more likely than those who did not to take gifts to prescribe more medications, more expensive medications, and more brand-name drugs (Wood et al., 2017). Although voluntary rules are in place to limit the relationships with and gifts from pharmaceutical companies, sample medications provided at the clinic by a company's representative and educational programs continue to influence practitioners.

One of the most challenging aspects to prescribing can occur when patients have strong, erroneous, or unrealistic beliefs about their care. Some patients may be demanding, complaining, or rude, and require more extensive interaction than other patients. While these situations may prompt the label of "difficult patient," alternative terminology such as "difficult patient situations" or "complex patient interactions" is more appropriate. "Standing one's ground" with rational prescribing can be difficult in the face of patients' demands for specific medications such as antibiotics. How can the APRN handle situations in which the patient assumes an adversarial role? Chapter 6, Managing Difficult and Complex Patient Interactions, has a full discussion of this topic. There are times, however, when a patient's specific medication request may be appropriate to consider. For example, when the next step in treatment of depression is medication, a patient may request the specific drug a family member had success with. Provided there are no contraindications to that specific drug and there is not a superior option, working with the patient's preference can build rapport.

SPECIAL CONSIDERATIONS FOR PRESCRIBING
Overview

APRNs have clinical competencies to provide healthcare for diverse populations in diverse settings which include emergency departments, primary care clinics, retail clinics, extended care facilities, prisons, and hospitals. APRNs also work in specialties such as oncology, geriatrics, dermatology, rheumatology, orthopedics, nephrology, cardiology, and palliative care. The prescribing role will be influenced by factors such as national certification and licensure, the population focus or specialization, the setting, and the community.

Prescribing for specific populations

Many psychiatric mental health NPs work with children. There are few medications approved by the FDA for use with children with mental health problems including depression, bipolar disorder, and schizophrenia. Conversely, there is an abundance of CSs marketed to treat children with attention deficit hyperactivity disorder (ADHD). This may lead parents to request these medications for behavioral issues even if the APRN does not diagnose ADHD.

The neonatal, pediatric, and family NP and pediatric CNSs may prescribe medication for children. Prescription challenges in this population sometimes involve calculating doses based on weight. As a vulnerable population, there is limited research on medication use in children. Consequently, a great deal of prescribing for children is not FDA approved and is known as "off label." Factors such as size, age, renal function, cardiac output, hepatic blood flow, and genetics affect pharmacokinetics and pharmacodynamics among children. Pediatric prescribing must consider various factors such as absorption of drugs, drug distribution, drug metabolism, and drug elimination (Garzon Maaks et al., 2020). Over-the-counter medications for children pose potential risks. Cold and cough preparations have not been adequately studied and are not recommended for children younger than six years of age (Lowry & Leeder, 2015). For example, excessive acetaminophen is associated with hepatic toxicity and use of aspirin during a viral infection may induce Reyes syndrome. It is critical therefore to routinely educate parents about seeking APRN guidance before using over-the-counter medications with children.

Adult gerontology primary and acute care NPs often work with patients who have polypharmacy complicated by mental and physical deficits. Polypharmacy increases the complexity of therapy, increases costs, and increases the risk of adverse consequences. As previously noted, use of the Beers Criteria and the STOPP screening tool can enhance rational prescribing.

The types of drugs that CRNAs order and administer have potentially serious and immediate consequences. For example, when propofol is used for sedation, the CRNA must be alert to the rapid onset of action, which is often within a minute. This rapid onset is dose-dependent and can result in an impaired respiratory drive, cause apnea, and require airway management.

CNMs, CNSs, and NPs must constantly consider the potential teratogenic effects of drugs in pregnant women. They must also consider the safety of drugs in lactating women. There are few randomized controlled trials regarding the safety of medications during pregnancy and lactation. To address this, the safety of medications is rated based on what information is available. Often the safety of a drug is unknown, and the APRN must proceed with caution and respond with evidence to the patient about her perception of risks and benefits.

NPs, CNSs, and CRNAs who work in pain management and palliative care typically prescribe a wide variety of CSs. Pain management requires expertise both in selecting medications and in dealing with patients who request medications that may not be indicated. Compliance with state laws implemented to deal with the US opioid crisis is imperative to assure patient safety and protect the APRN's license (see Chapter 7). In contrast, APRNs who work with patients in palliative care may need to provide education to dispel concerns about opioid addiction at the end of life.

Other special considerations

An employer or health system may restrict APRN prescribing more than the law does. The VA and health maintenance organizations such as Kaiser Permanente use preferred drug lists, or formularies, to promote evidence-based prescribing and control costs. Similarly, Medicaid and Medicare set guidelines for drug benefits, while private health plans usually have different tiers of drug coverage to promote prescribing of effective lowest cost drugs.

Pharmacy benefit managers are another aspect of the medication distribution chain, negotiating with drug companies and pharmacies on behalf of health plans. They develop formularies on behalf of the health plans, negotiate discounts and rebates with the manufacturers, and contract with pharmacies to reimburse for drugs dispensed to health plan beneficiaries (Commonwealth Fund, 2019). Some retailers have drugs dispensed for reduced costs, such as a $4 or $10 prescription, or offer reduced rates based on membership (Torrey, 2019). Discount coupons are often available from the manufacturer for some high-cost medications or discount programs.

THE FUTURE OF THE APRN PRESCRIBING ROLE

The US opioid epidemic, increasing antibiotic resistance, the escalating costs of prescription drugs, and limited access to medication in under resourced countries are a few examples of why rational prescribing is imperative. A balance between pharmacological and non-pharmacological treatment options is becoming increasingly desirable as many patients use herbal remedies and supplements and seek more holistic healing approaches, choosing to avoid medication risks and side effects. New scientific information may also reveal additional considerations about medication safety or sequelae. The APRN has the opportunity to meet these demands using evidence-based practices and rational prescribing. As the evidence base for pharmacological treatment changes and the use of electronic prescribing increases, the APRN must adapt prescribing practices. Adoption of the prescriber role is a career-long process that requires vigilance and wisdom.

REFERENCES

Abramson, E. (2015). Causes and consequences of e-prescribing errors in community pharmacies. *Integrated Pharmacy Research and Practice, 4*(5), 31–38.

Agency for Healthcare Research and Quality. (2020) Medication errors and adverse drug events. Retrieved from https://psnet.ahrq.gov/primer/medication-errors-and-adverse-drug-events. (Accessed 7 September 2020.)

Alabama State Board of Nursing. (2020). Nurse Practice Act Article 5, Advanced Practice Nursing §34-21-86. Retrieved from https://www.abn.alabama.gov/wp-content/uploads/2016/02/nursing-practice-act-article-5.pdf. (Accessed 7 September 2020.)

Alex, S., Adenew, A.B., Arundel, C., et al. (2016). Medication errors despite using electronic health records: The value of a clinical pharmacist service in reducing discharge-related medication errors. *Quality Management in Health Care, 25*(1), 32–37.

Blanco-Reina, E., Arixza-Zafra, G., Ocana-Ricola, R., & Leon-Ortiz, M. (2014). 2012 American Geriatrics Society Beers Criteria: Enhanced applicability for detecting potentially inappropriate medications in European older adults? A comparison with the Screening Tool of Older Person's Potentially Inappropriate Prescriptions. *Journal of the American Geriatric Society, 62*(7), 1217–1223.

Brown, S.A., & Grimes, D.E. (1995). A meta-analysis of nurse practitioners and nurse midwives in primary care. *Nursing Research, 44*(6), 332–339.

Brown, M.A., & Olshansky, E. (1998). Becoming a primary care nurse practitioner: Challenges of the initial year of practice. *Nurse Practitioner, 23*(7), 46, 52–56, 58.

Brykcznski, K.A. (2019). Role development of the advanced practice nurse. In M.F. Tracy & E.T. O'Grady (Eds), *Hamric and Hanson's advanced practice nursing: an integrative approach* (6th ed., pp. 80–108). St. Louis, MO: Saunders Elsevier Health Sciences.

Code of Colorado Regulations. (2017). Board of nursing. 3CCR 716-1. (1.15) rules and regulations for prescriptive authority for advanced practice registered nurses. Retrieved from https://www.sos.state.co.us/CCR/GenerateRulePdf.do?ruleVersionId=9035&fileName=3%20CCR%20716-1. (Accessed 2 November 2020.)

Commonwealth Fund. (2019). Pharmacy benefit managers and their role ion drug spending. Retrieved from https://www.commonwealthfund.org/publications/explainer/2019/apr/pharmacy-benefit-managers-and-their-role-drug-spending. (Accessed 7 September 2020.)

Congressional Budget Office. (1979). *Physician extenders: Their current and future role in medical care delivery.* Washington, DC: US Government Printing Office.

DeFrank, J.T., Berkman, N.D., Kahwathi, L., et al. (2019). Direct-to-consumer advertising of prescription drugs and the patient–prescriber encounter: A systematic review. *Health Communication, 35*(6), 739–146.

DesRoches, C.M., Clarke, S., Perloff, J., et al. (2017). The quality of primary care provided by nurse practitioners to vulnerable Medicare beneficiaries. *Nursing Outlook, 65*(6), 679–688.

Dulisse, B., & Cromwell, J. (2010). No harm found when nurse anesthetists work without supervision by physicians. *Health Affairs, 29*(8), 1469–1475.

Dunphy, L.M. (2018). Advanced practice nursing: Doing what has to be done. In L. Joel (Ed.), *Advanced practice nursing: Essentials for role development* (pp. 2–16). Philadelphia: F.A. Davis.

Farrell, V.M., Hill, V.L., Hawkins, J.B., et al. (2003). Clinic for identifying and addressing polypharmacy. *American Journal of Health-System Pharmacy, 60*(18), 1834–1835.

Fick, D.M., Cooper, J.W., Wade, W.E., et al. (2003). Updating the Beers Criteria for potentially inappropriate medication use in older adults: Results of a US consensus panel of experts. *Archives of Internal Medicine, 163*(22), 2716–2724.

Filipova, A. (2019). Relationship of direct-to-consumer advertising to efficiency of care, quality of care and health outcomes. *Journal for Healthcare Quality, 42*(3), e18–e31.

Fletcher, C.E., Baker, S.J., Copeland, L.A., et al. (2007). Nurse practitioners' and physicians' views of NPs as providers of primary care to veterans. *Journal of Nursing Scholarship, 39*(4), 358–362.

Fulton, M.M., & Allen, E.R. (2005). Polypharmacy in the elderly: A literature review. *Journal of the American Academy of Nurse Practitioners, 17*(4), 123–132.

Garzon Maaks, D.L., Starr, N.B., Brady, M.A., et al. (2020). *Burns' pediatric primary care* (7th ed.). St. Louis, MO: Elsevier.

Grace, P.J. (2009). *Nursing ethics and professional responsibility in advanced practice.* Sudbury, MA: Jones & Bartlett.

Horrocks, S., Anderson, E., & Salisbury, C. (2002). Systematic review of whether nurse practitioners working in primary care can provide equivalent care to doctors. *British Medical Journal, 324*(7341), 819–823.

Jennings, N., Clifford, S., Fox, A.R., et al. (2015). The impact of nurse practitioner services on cost, quality of care, satisfaction and waiting times in the emergency department: A systematic review. *International Journal of Nursing Studies 52*(1), 421–435.

Jones, L.K., Ladd, I.G., Gregor, C., et al. (2019). Understanding the medication prior-authorization process: A case study of patients and clinical staff from a large rural integrated health delivery system. *American Journal of Health Systems Pharmacy, 76*(7), 453–459.

Kaplan, L., & Brown, M.A. (2004). Prescriptive authority and barriers to NP practice. *The Nurse Practitioner, 29*(3), 28–35.

Kaplan, L., & Brown, M.A. (2006). What is "true" professional autonomy? *Nurse Practitioner, 31*(3), 37.

Kraus, E., & DuBois, J.M. (2017). Knowing your limits: A qualitative study of physician and nurse practitioner perspectives of NP independence in primary care. *Journal of General Internal Medicine, 32*(3), 284–290.

Landsperger, J.S., Semler, M.W., Wang, L., et al. (2016). Outcomes of nurse practitioner-delivered critical care: A prospective cohort study. *Chest, 149*(5), 1146–1154.

Laurant, M., van der Biezen, M., Wijers, N., et al. (2018). Nurses as substitutes for doctors in primary care. *Cochrane Database Systematic Reviews, 7*(7), CD001271.

Lenz, E.R., Mundinger, M.O., Kane, R.L., et al. (2004). Primary care outcomes in patients treated by nurse practitioners or physicians: two year follow up. *Medical Care Research and Review, 51*(3), 332–351.

Lowry, J.A., & Leeder, J.S. (2015). Over-the-counter medications: Update on cough and cold preparations. *Pediatrics in Review, 36*(7), 286–298.

McVeigh, D.M. (2001). Polypharmacy in the older population: Recommendations for improved clinical practice. *Topics in Emergency Medicine, 23*(3), 68–75.

National Council of State Boards of Nursing. (2020). Member board profiles. Retrieved from https://www.ncsbn.org/profiles.htm. (Accessed 7 September 2020.)

National Conference of State Legislatures. (2020). State medical marijuana laws. Retrieved from http://www.ncsl.org/research/health/state-medical-marijuana-laws.aspx. (Accessed 7 September 2020.)

Newhouse, R.P., Stanik-Hutt, J., White, K.M., et al. (2011). Advance practice nurse outcomes 1990–2008: A systematic review. *Nursing Economics, 29*(5), 1–22.

Ohman-Strickland, P.A., Orzano, A.J., Hudson, S.V., et al. (2008). Quality of diabetes care in family medicine practices: Influence of nurse practitioners and physician's assistants. *Annals of Family Medicine, 6*(1), 14–22.

O'Keefe, M.E. (2001). *Nursing practice and the law.* Philadelphia: F.A. Davis Company.

Phillips, S.J. (2007). A comprehensive look at the legislative issues affecting advanced nursing practice. *The Nurse Practitioner, 32*(1), 14–17.

Prescott, P.A., & Driscoll, L. (1980). Evaluating nurse practitioner performance. *Nurse Practitioner, 1*(1), 28–32.

Safriet, B.J. (1992). Health care dollars and regulatory sense: The role of advanced practice nursing. *Yale Journal on Regulation, 9*(2), 417–488.

Safriet, B.J. (2002). Closing the gap between can and may in healthcare provider's scopes of practice: A primer for policymakers. *Yale Journal on Regulation, 19*(2), 301–334.

Schommer, J.C., Worley, M.M., Kjos, A.L., et al. (2009). A thematic analysis for how patients, prescribers, experts, and patient advocates view the prescription choice process. *Research in Social and Administrative Pharmacy, 5*(2), 154–169.

Schumacher, K.L., & Meleis, A.I. (1994). Transitions: A central concept in nursing. *Image: The Journal of Nursing Scholarship, 26*(2), 119–127.

Simonson, D.C., Ahern, M.M., & Hendryx, M.S. (2007). Anesthesia staffing and anesthetic complications during cesarean delivery: A retrospective analysis. *Nursing Research, 56*(1), 9–17.

Spitzer, W.O., Sackett, D.L., Sibley, J.C., et al. (1974). The Burlington randomized trial of the nurse practitioner. *New England Journal of Medicine, 290*(3), 252–256.

Title 21 – Food and Drugs. (1993). 21 USC Chapter 13, subchapter I, Part B, 1993: Authority to control; standards and schedules. Retrieved from https://uscode.house.gov/view.xhtml?path=/prelim@title21/chapter13/subchapter1/partB&edition=prelim. (Accessed 7 September 2020.)

Torrey, T. (2019). Where to find free or low-cost prescription drugs. *Very Well Health*. Retrieved from https://www.verywellhealth.com/free-low-cost-prescription-drugs-stores-2615299. (Accessed 7 September 2020.)

Ulrich, C.M., & Soeken, K. (2005). A path analytic model of ethical conflict in practice and autonomy in a sample of nurse practitioners. *Nursing Ethics, 12*(3), 319–325.

Washington State Health Care Authority. (2020). Patient review and coordination program. Retrieved from https://www.hca.wa.gov/billers-providers-partners/programs-and-services/patient-review-and-coordination-prc. (Accessed 7 September 2020.)

Weiland, S.A. (2008). Reflections on independence in nurse practitioner practice. *Journal of the American Academy of Nurse Practitioners, 20*(7), 345–352.

Weiland, S.A. (2015). Understanding nurse practitioner autonomy. *Journal of the American Association of Nurse Practitioners, 27*(2), 95–104.

Wood, S.F., Podrasky, J., McMonagle, M.A., et al. (2017). Influence of pharmaceutical marketing on Medicare prescriptions in the District of Columbia. *PLoS One, 12*(10), e0186060.

World Health Organization. (2002). Promoting rational use of medicines: Core components. WHO Policy Perspectives on Medicines. Retrieved from http://archives.who.int/tbs/rational/h3011e.pdf. (Accessed 7 September 2020.)

Wright, W.L., Romboli, J.E., DiTulio, M.A., et al. (2011). Hypertension treatment and control within an independent nurse practitioner setting. *American Journal of Managed Care, 17*(1), 58–65.

Creating a Practice Environment for Full Prescriptive Authority

3

Louise Kaplan and Marie Annette Brown

This chapter focuses on the range of external and internal barriers that can affect advanced practice registered nurses (APRNs) as prescribers. External factors are generally a part of the practice environment and include factors such as laws, regulations, and policies, as well as the attitudes of other health professionals. Internal barriers are invisible or unacknowledged factors within the individual APRN, including personal characteristics such as conflict avoidance or the "need to be liked." Strategies to overcome internal and external prescribing barriers are offered as a way to generate enthusiasm among APRNs for facilitating change.

Advanced practice registered nurses (APRNs) confront a multitude of opportunities and challenges when prescribing medications. Some opportunities and challenges result from laws, regulations, and policies that either promote or limit prescribing and are external to the individual. Other factors intrinsic to the individual, such as attitudes toward prescribing specific medications, may also promote or limit APRN prescribing. The external and internal factors described in this chapter limit prescribing and serve as barriers that significantly restrict the potential for fully autonomous practice, the ultimate vision of APRNs.

Some APRNs work tirelessly to eliminate factors that create external and internal barriers to practice. Other APRNs do not perceive these factors as barriers and accept reduced and restricted practice environments. Research in Washington State during a transition to a new scope of practice suggests that "NPs in most states accepted physician control or supervision as a 'first step' in order to have any legal authorization to practice. Over the years, however, many NPs have accepted restrictions in autonomy which become normalized as 'good enough.' It may be easier for some NPs to maintain the status quo than to adopt a new scope of practice" (Kaplan & Brown, 2008, p. 52). The fear that "making waves" could diminish job security and the cost of obtaining Drug Enforcement Administration (DEA) registration are common examples reported in studies as deterrents to transitioning to more autonomous practice (Kaplan et al., 2006). A core value that needs to be cultivated in APRN

The Advanced Practice Registered Nurse as a Prescriber, Second Edition. Edited by Louise Kaplan and Marie Annette Brown.

education and practice is commitment to actively work toward the goal of full practice authority nationwide.

Both external and internal barriers to prescribing medications are equally important to understand and to be addressed. Any prescribing barrier, no matter how small, affects the ability of APRNs to practice to the full extent of their education and license. Given the demands of practice in a complex healthcare system, it is critical to eliminate barriers to prescribing and attain the goal of creating a national practice environment for full practice authority.

EXTERNAL BARRIERS TO PRESCRIBING
Federal laws and policies

Although states provide most regulation of prescriptive authority, the federal government affects certain aspects of prescribing. The most significant aspect is regulation of prescribing controlled substances (CSs). Any healthcare professional who prescribes Schedule II–V medications must register with the DEA or work for a healthcare organization that has institutional DEA registration. Prescribing, dispensing, and administering scheduled drugs are regulated by the Controlled Substances Act of 1970 (Title 21 – Food and Drugs, 1970).

Some federal laws that restrict prescribing affect all healthcare professionals. For example, federal law requires that methadone, when used for opioid dependence, be administered or dispensed, but not prescribed, to patients only in licensed Opioid Treatment Programs (OTPs) (Public Health Service, 2018). Federal law also stipulates: "OTPs must ensure that opioid agonist treatment medications are administered or dispensed only by a practitioner licensed under the appropriate State law and registered under the appropriate State and Federal laws to administer or dispense opioid drugs, or by an agent of such a practitioner, supervised by and under the order of the licensed practitioner" (Public Health Service, 2018, p. 105). Prescribers may, however, prescribe methadone for pain management.

The Drug Addiction Treatment Act (2000) authorized only qualifying physicians to prescribe buprenorphine in the office-based setting. The Comprehensive Addiction and Recovery Act of 2016 added nurse practitioners (NPs) to the definition of qualifying providers who could prescribe medications in the office-based setting but only until October 1, 2021 (Public Law 114-198, 2016). In 2018 Congress passed the Substance Use-Disorder Prevention that Promotes Opioid Recovery and Treatment for Patients and Communities Act which made permanent the addition of nurse practitioners as qualifying practitioners (Public Law 115-271, 2018). The law also added certified nurse midwives (CNMs), certified registered nurse anesthetists (CRNAs), and clinical nurse specialists (CNSs) as qualifying practitioners; however, they were authorized only until October 1, 2023. The law regulates the required training to be eligible for a DEA waiver to prescribe office-based medication assisted treatment (MAT) and the number of patients a provider may treat.

Some federal laws that affect APRN prescribing are not always as obvious as those related to CSs. Medicare is the government-administered health plan for people aged 65 and older and some people with disabilities. Not until 2020 with congressional passage of the Coronavirus Aid, Relief, and Economic Security Act could NPs and CNSs document home health face-to-face assessments and certify and recertify a patient's eligibility for home health. This applies to Medicaid programs as well

(Public Law 116-136, 2020). The law did not apply to hospices. As well, APRNs are prohibited from ordering diabetic shoes, offering cardiac and pulmonary rehabilitation, and providing several other therapies for Medicare patients.

State laws and rules

All states authorize NPs and CNMs to prescribe, order, or furnish medications. Some states, however, do not authorize CNSs or CRNAs to prescribe. Only 36 states and the District of Columbia (DC) authorize CNSs to prescribe, while 37 states and DC authorize CRNAs to prescribe (National Council of State Boards of Nursing [NCSBN], 2020).

Even though all states authorize NPs to prescribe, order, or furnish medications, only DC and 25 states (the number varies depending on the definition) have full practice authority. Some states require use of a formulary or protocol, or prescribing based on the agreement with or delegation by a physician for either a designated period of time or career-long (NCSBN, 2020). The state of Georgia serves as the quintessential example of restricted practice. Georgia allows prescribing only as a delegated authority and the law is explicit that "ordering" a drug shall not be construed as prescribing. Box 3.1 is a section of the Georgia rules

---

Box 3.1 Georgia Board of Nursing selected rules on APRN prescriptive authority

Rule 410-11-14 Regulation of Protocol Use by Advanced Practice Registered Nurses as Authorized by O.C.G.A. Section 43-34-26.3

(2) An APRN may practice under a nurse protocol agreement authorized by O.C.G.A. § 43-34-25 if the nurse protocol agreement adheres to the following criteria . . .

(e) Shall comply with the provisions of O.C.G.A. § 43-34-26.3 regarding prescription drug orders placed by an APRN for a drug or medical device including, but not limited to, the following:

1. No prescription drug orders submitted by an APRN for Schedule I or II controlled substances;
2. No refills of any drug for more than 12 months from the date of the original order, except in the case of oral contraceptives, hormone replacement therapy, or prenatal vitamins, which may be refilled for a period of 24 months;
3. No drug order or medical device that may result in the performance or occurrence of an abortion, including the administration, prescription, or issuance of a drug order that is intended to cause an abortion to occur pharmacologically;
4. Written prescription drug orders shall be signed by the APRN, be written on forms that comply with the nurse protocol agreement, and such forms shall contain the information required by paragraph (d) of O.C.G.A. §43-34-26.3;
5. A written provision in the nurse protocol agreement authorizing the APRN to request, receive, and sign for professional samples, and to distribute them to patients in accordance with a list of professional samples approved by the delegating physician that is maintained by the office or facility where the APRN works and that requires the documentation of each sample received and dispensed; and
6. Compliance with applicable state and federal laws and regulations pertaining to the ordering, maintenance, and dispensing of drugs.

Source: From Georgia Comprehensive Rules & Regulations, 2019. © Lawriter LLC. Reprinted with permissions of Lawriter LLC.

Box 3.2 Georgia Composite Board of Medicine rules on APRN prescriptive authority

§43-34-25. Delegation of certain medical acts to advanced practice registered nurse; construction and limitations of such delegation; definitions; conditions of nurse protocol; issuance of prescription drug orders.

A nurse protocol agreement between a physician and an advanced practice registered nurse pursuant to this Code section shall: . . .

(c) (9) Provide that a patient who receives a prescription drug order for any controlled substance pursuant to a nurse protocol agreement shall be evaluated or examined by the delegating physician or other physician designated by the delegating physician pursuant to paragraph (2) of this subsection on at least a quarterly basis or at a more frequent interval as determined by the board.

(d) A written prescription drug order issued pursuant to this Code Section shall be signed by the advanced practice registered nurse and shall be on a form which shall include, without limitation, the names of the advanced practice registered nurse and delegating physician who are parties to the nurse protocol agreement, the patient's name and address, the drug or device ordered, directions with regard to the taking and dosage of the drug or use of the device, and the number of refills. A prescription drug order which is transmitted either electronically or via facsimile shall conform to the requirements set out in paragraphs (1) and (2) of subsection (c) of Code Section 26-4-80, respectively.

(e) An APRN may be authorized under a nurse protocol agreement to request, receive, and sign for professional samples and may distribute professional samples to patients . . ..

Source: From Code of Georgia, 2019. Public Domain.

---

authorizing APRNs to place prescription drug orders under a nurse protocol agreement with a physician approved by the Georgia Board of Medicine. As a delegated act, the Georgia Medical Practice Act must also be referenced to have complete information about what is required for the APRN to order medications. Box 3.2 is one relevant section of the Georgia Medical Practice Act.

Another type of prescribing restriction occurs in California where qualified NPs are issued a furnishing number to "order" or furnish drugs and devices according to approved standardized procedure or protocol. Prior to receiving a furnishing number, a certified NP must complete both an approved pharmacology course and a minimum of 520 hours of physician-supervised experience furnishing drugs and/or devices (California Business and Professions Code, 2019). Some restrictions may seem minor, but when they exist in law, they must be followed and serve as barriers because they limit full autonomy. In Utah, the law stipulates that an APRN who prescribes Schedule II and III CSs must do so in accordance with a consultation and referral plan (Utah Nurse Practice Act, 2013).

In states that require collaborative agreements or supervision for APRN prescribing, there are sometimes limits to the number of APRNs physicians can supervise. South Carolina allows a physician to supervise no more than six full-time equivalent APRNs (Phillips, 2020), while Texas physicians may delegate prescribing or ordering a drug or device to no more than seven, or seven full-time-equivalent, APRNs and physician assistants (PAs) (Texas Administrative Code, 2013). Florida limits physician supervision to an unspecified number, instead stipulating that the limit should assure an acceptable standard of medical care is rendered (Florida Administrative Code & Florida Administrative Register, 2017).

Legal authorization to prescribe CSs is one of the underpinnings of fully autonomous practice. There is wide variation among the APRN roles regarding which ones can prescribe CSs. CRNAs do not have CS prescriptive authority in 16 states, CNMs do not have it in 3 states, and CNSs do not have it in 13 states (NCSBN, 2020). NPs in Alabama have no authority through the Board of Nursing to prescribe CSs. They must apply to the Alabama Board of Medical Examiners to secure a controlled drug certificate protocol that has several requirements for eligibility, including 12 months of active clinical practice once granted an approved collaborative practice agreement (Alabama Board of Nursing, 2019).

Kentucky is an example of a state with many constraints on CS prescribing. CS II medications may be prescribed only for a 72-hour supply without refills with two exceptions. CS II hydrocodone combination products may be prescribed for up to a 30-day supply with no refills. Psychostimulants may be prescribed by psychiatric/mental health APRNs who work in certain types of facilities for a 30-day supply. Schedule III prescriptions are limited to a 30-day supply, while Schedule IV and V drugs may be prescribed with up to six refills (Kentucky Revised Statutes, 2018). Exceptions in Schedule IV are prescriptions for diazepam (Valium®), clonazepam (Klonopin®), lorazepam (Ativan®), alprazolam (Xanax®), and carisprodol (Soma®) which are limited to a 30-day supply without refills (Kentucky Administrative Regulations, 2013).

In addition to the state laws and regulations that govern APRN prescribing, states sometimes have additional laws and rules that apply to all prescribers, especially related to CSs. While these are not specific to APRNs, the state laws still present another hurdle that can require time and effort, and cause confusion. For example, the federal Controlled Substances Act does not set an expiration date for a CS II prescription (Drug Enforcement Administration, 2006). In Nebraska, however, a Schedule II prescription may not be dispensed by a pharmacist more than six months from the date it was issued (Nebraska Revised Statute, 2017). Some states require a special permit to prescribe CSs in addition to DEA registration. Connecticut requires that any practitioner authorized to prescribe, administer, and dispense CSs obtain a Connecticut Controlled Substance Registration prior to applying for DEA registration (Connecticut General Assembly, 2013). Problems also arise when states prohibit or restrict pharmacists from dispensing medication prescribed by APRNs from another state. In Texas, prescriptions from APRNs in other states may be filled with the exception of CSs, even though a Texas APRN may prescribe CSs (Texas State Board of Pharmacy, 2019).

Other barriers

Despite removal of federal law as a barrier to APRN prescribing buprenorphine for MAT, other barriers exist. Among respondents to a survey, NPs and PAs prescribing MAT reported barriers including concerns about diversion and misuse, lack of mental health or psychosocial support services, lack of specialty backup for complex problems, and time constraints. Even though some NPs and PAs are authorized to prescribe MAT, they do not utilize the authority. These providers noted that key barriers were clinic policies, resistance from practice colleagues, and lack of specialty backup (Andrilla et al., 2019).

In response to the US opioid epidemic, states have provided voluntary evidence-based recommendations and implemented a variety of laws to reduce the number of opioid prescriptions for acute, subacute, and chronic noncancer. In 2016, Massachusetts passed a law that limits opioid prescriptions to a seven-day supply. Subsequently, over 30 more states have laws that set limits on, provide guidance, or specify requirements for opioid prescriptions (National Conference of State Legislatures, 2019). Prescription drug monitoring programs (PDMPs) enable NPs to objectively assess a patient's use of CSs. In some states, use of the PDMP is required prior to providing a prescription for an initial or refill of a CS by some or all prescribers (Pew Charitable Trusts, 2018).

INTERNAL BARRIERS TO PRESCRIBING

Internal barriers are often unacknowledged factors within the individual APRN and can be overlooked when analyzing barriers to APRN prescribing. For example, lack of expertise to prescribe a specific medication or class of medications and the time required to obtain this information are internal barriers. For CSs, internal barriers may include aversion to patients perceived to have drug-seeking behaviors and/or the responsibility of prescribing CSs.

Internal barriers may arise when APRN education does not include the full range of prescribing competencies. Role socialization may also contribute to the development of internal barriers. Professional attitudes and values are developed through the educational environment, interactions with other healthcare professionals, and community practice norms. These attitudes and values shape an individual's approach to prescribing and contribute to the development of a full range of prescribing competencies.

Prescribing competencies must include the ability to effectively communicate with patients in challenging clinical situations. Patients may request specific medications such as antibiotics, CSs, or brand-name drugs they identify from direct-to-consumer advertising. APRNs may have a variety of reactions to these requests ranging from resistance to acquiescence to acceptance. Skillful APRN prescribers can help patients and families understand what types of medications are and are not appropriate for particular situations. An exemplar of national efforts to assist all prescribers with these challenges is the Centers for Disease Control and Prevention's program using evidence-based guidelines to promote judicious antibiotic prescribing. "Be Antibiotics Aware" has resources for the public and healthcare professionals.

Another issue, resistance to prescribing CSs, may stem from the APRN's perception that the patient is exhibiting "drug-seeking behavior." This assumption may or may not be correct because some patients are simply attempting to adequately manage their health needs. Requests for widely advertised, brand-name drugs are common. Information alone about the equivalency of generic and brand-name drugs and the cost differential may or may not change patient preferences. Prescribing decisions are ideally made based on a patient-centered approach and "knowing the patient" to tailor the discussion in light of the patient's decision-making approaches. These situations emphasize the importance of skills such as motivational interviewing.

Prescribing CSs may evoke a constellation of concerns that prompt some APRNs to avoid the responsibilities associated with these drugs particularly in respect to the opioid epidemic and overprescribing of opioid medications. These concerns include issues such as the potential for patient addiction or diversion and APRN fear of legal or disciplinary action. Knowledge of state laws and policies previously noted regarding responsible opioid prescribing is imperative and can allay the prescriber's anxiety if they adhere to guidelines. It is also essential to be aware of changes in approaches to assessment of pain and standards for pain management when considering the need for a CS prescription. For example, the Joint Commission's reference to pain as the "fifth vital sign" was misinterpreted as a commission standard rather than as a phrase to bring attention to the need for improved pain assessment. By 2004 the Commission eliminated reference to "the fifth vital sign" in its accreditation standards, and in all of its materials several years later (Baker, 2017). Nonetheless, pain assessment is often conducted routinely even if not related to the presenting problem. Meanwhile, many providers limit or do not provide care for pain management. Patients who do experience chronic pain are sometimes not provided with prescriptions due to clinics adopting no-opioid policies, forcing an end to long-term provider–patient relationships.

Development of prescribing competencies through appropriate education and training provides the essential foundation for practice. The early decades of NP role development provided few opportunities for identifying and implementing prescribing competencies. The current healthcare environment presents daunting challenges from the overwhelming amount of information necessary for competent prescribing. Lack of knowledge about a specific drug or class of medications is an internal barrier that may limit an APRN's ability to provide comprehensive care. APRNs may describe this situation by stating they have "no need" for specific medications or that they are not comfortable or competent in a specific area of prescribing.

At the same time, it is essential that APRNs prescribe within the scope of their practice and their knowledge base. Self-assessment of limitations is central to safe, quality practice. It is also important to emphasize that providers are not responsible for prescribing every class of medication. Professional autonomy provides the foundation for each APRN to create an individualized approach to safe, quality practice.

Another important aspect of internal barriers relates to the APRN's sense of autonomy. State laws, community standards, and practice policies may lead to a limited perspective among some APRNs and other health professionals about APRN autonomous prescribing. Over time, norms often develop that perpetuate acceptance of these restrictions. In Washington State, which has had independent practice authorized since 1973 and full prescriptive authority since 2005, only 83% of respondents to an APRN survey in 2006 reported that they felt fully autonomous (Kaplan et al., 2010). Ambivalence about autonomous practice and prescribing as well as the willingness to accept practice limitations serve as internal barriers to autonomous prescribing.

STRATEGIES TO ADDRESS PRESCRIBING BARRIERS

The elimination of both external and internal barriers is vitally important to attain full prescriptive authority nationwide. Change requires proactive strategies on multiple levels. Strategies to promote fully autonomous prescribing include a range of actions – from individual self-assessment and reflection to lobbying for changes to state or federal law. Development and implementation of these strategies requires consideration of the sociocultural context and prescribing environments, which vary widely across the nation. For example, cultural norms and gender politics about women's access to power and self-determination are limited in some communities. Consequently, APRNs need to utilize state-specific approaches with their advocacy to change restrictive laws and practices.

Legislative activities, regulatory change, and advocacy contribute to the elimination of external prescribing barriers. Little attention, however, has been paid to internal barriers. Some APRNs may normalize a supervised or constrained environment or report "no need" to expand their scope of practice. An individual or small group of APRNs who understand the local and broader need for APRNs' full practice authority can "raise the consciousness" of their practice colleagues and champion changes in their individual setting. Often, a key first step is bringing together the APRNs in a practice or organization to obtain a fuller picture of the constrained APRN practice environment. A deeper understanding of the advantages of "what might be possible" can strengthen APRNs' commitment to change. Local, state, and national professional groups and organizations can be a source of evidence-based, well-designed literature advocating the benefits of fully autonomous APRN practice to patients and the healthcare systems. It is also essential for APRN faculty to prepare the next generation of APRNs with the expectation of full practice authority. Faculty can strengthen curriculum that develops students' skills and commitment to initiate change if complacency exists in their new practice environment. New graduates who understand their responsibility to change can inspire colleagues with their enthusiasm. Faculty and student commitment to this vision can help build expertise to implement strategies that facilitate readiness for change to full practice authority.

ELIMINATING EXTERNAL BARRIERS TO PRESCRIBING
Legislative activities

Each state's Nurse Practice Act (NPA) generally defines APRN scope of practice, although several states involve the Board of Medicine or other entities. The NPA is created by legislators who often lack a deep understanding of APRN expertise. Consequently, it is important to develop a cadre of politically competent APRNs who can serve as consultants to policymakers and their staff. Relationships with legislators provide the foundation to encourage them to become sponsors and champions of bills that improve APRN scope of practice, including autonomous prescribing. Success in passing APRN legislation may require years of lobbying to educate legislators and gain their support. Success is sometimes incremental. Several states have improved their practice environment from restricted practice to reduced practice or created a process for transition to full practice authority after a period of years in collaborative practice with a physician or APRN (Phillips, 2020).

Effective lobbying results from strong nursing organizations and creation of coalitions among APRNs. As APRN and public interests are usually aligned, it is important for APRNs to participate in public discourse on health policy issues. APRNs can utilize their expertise to support legislation that promotes access to care, encourages reduction of health disparities, and enhances quality patient care. Box 3.3 recommends a strategy to educate policymakers about the benefits of APRN practice and highlights information necessary for this process. Box 3.4 provides an overview of the key elements involved in lobbying for legislative changes.

Box 3.3 Recommendation: educate policymakers about the benefits of APRN practice

While APRNs are educated to provide comprehensive care, legal and policy restrictions continue to limit their practice. As the population ages and healthcare problems become increasingly complex, restrictive practice environments lead to the underutilization of APRN skills, knowledge, and abilities. Ultimately, policymakers need to formulate laws and regulations that result in autonomous practice to improve access to evidenced-based quality patient care provided by APRNs. Information needed to educate policymakers on the importance of fully autonomous APRN practice includes:

- The skills, knowledge, and abilities of APRNs
- Databased analyses of the outcomes of APRN care
- The influence of full practice authority on APRN practice and access to patient care.

In addition, APRNs should:
- Develop fact sheets about the quality and safety of APRN care
- Evaluate the "cost" of restrictions on APRN practice to the patient, the insurer, and society.

Box 3.4 Influencing legislative change

Know how the process works
Consult your state government's website for an overview of the legislative process and contact information for legislators.

Make yourself the expert
Do your homework: know who the issue affects, what others feel about it, how it will influence future trends, and any other important contextual information to the issue at hand. Combining this with your own personal experience is the most effective information you can provide.

Get to know your legislators
You can contact your legislators in a number of ways:

- Personal visit. Call the office, introduce yourself and the issue you would like to discuss, and make an appointment for a visit. Be prepared for your discussion. Know what you want to say, be factual, and make your comments as brief and specific as you can. Be clear about what you are asking the legislator to do, such as sponsor or support a bill, oppose a bill, or contact a state agency on behalf of the issue about which you are concerned.
- Attend a town hall meeting. Most legislators conduct periodic town hall meetings at various locations in their district or by audio/visual technology.
- Write a letter or email. Make your message to the point, clear, and formal. Include your full contact information so the legislator can respond via email or letter.
- Testify before a committee. Be prepared to articulate your views and positions at a public hearing on an issue or bill.

Get to know legislative staff
Legislators rely heavily on professional staff for information gathering and analysis. They work on a wide range of issues and always appreciate new sources of clear and accurate information. Members of staff can also supply you with the most current information available.

Network with other citizens
Find out whether there are groups that share your concerns and establish a network or coalition. A group of concerned citizens can be more effective working together, rather than as separate individuals trying to accomplish the same goal.

Source: Adapted from Washington State Legislature. (n.d.). *A Citizen's Guide to Effective Legislative Participation*. Retrieved from http://leg.wa.gov/legislature/pages/effectiveparticipation.aspx. (Accessed 7 September 2020.)

Successful interactions in the policy arena require effective communication. Underlying principles for communication include the following:

- Use clear, thoughtful language that avoids jargon and presents one's expertise.
- Use accurate, evidence-based information to establish credibility.
- Describe a problem without complaint and provide a realistic solution.
- Articulate how an issue has relevance beyond nursing.

- Use examples from professional practice to move an issue from the abstract to the concrete and "make it real."
- Use professional language and approaches that maintain equanimity and composure. Avoid the use of language that is sarcastic, demeaning, and inflammatory even if confronted by proposals or positions that are inaccurate or debasing, or that diminish the contributions of APRNs.

Regulatory changes

Regulatory change involves development of rules that may be necessary to implement a law as well as to fulfill the legislative mandates of governmental agencies. For example, a state's law that authorizes prescriptive authority with physician involvement requires rules to specify the precise nature of that involvement. States have administrative procedures acts that delineate the legal process for creating rules and afford the opportunity for public participation. It is imperative that APRNs participate in the regulatory process which is equally important as passing laws. Often, "the devil is in the detail," and the rules and implementation directly affect each APRN's practice experience.

APRNs individually or through professional organizations need to ensure that they are apprised of proposed rules that need to be analyzed to determine their impact on APRN practice. Comments can be sent in writing or given as testimony at a hearing. For example, rules may be proposed in a state to require physician-supervised practice hours to qualify for autonomous prescribing. APRNs could oppose this rule by providing APRN prescribing competencies developed in educational programs and evidence from other states with fully autonomous prescribing.

Advocacy

Advocacy involves active support for a cause or position. Advocacy about the APRN role and competencies most often occurs during daily interactions with patients and colleagues. The need for advocacy, however, extends to a multitude of issues – from those in the workplace to national health policies. A great deal of advocacy occurs beyond the legislative and regulatory process, such as responding to misrepresentations of APRN practice by the American Medical Association; raising public awareness through media campaigns; community service to promote the APRN role; and participation in health-related and community advisory boards. Advocacy often occurs on an individual level, for example, sending a letter to the editor of a media outlet that publishes or reports an inaccurate or limited view of APRN practice. Advocacy can be direct or indirect. Membership in national APRN organizations supports their efforts to be a strong voice for APRNs on issues such as assuring provider neutral language in health policies. Local-level advocacy for provider neutral language is common when APRNs request their clinics and health systems demonstrate inclusiveness.

Prescribing-related advocacy provides an opportunity for APRNs to contribute to health policy at multiple levels. APRNs can challenge pharmaceutical companies to change package labeling and marketing materials to use the term healthcare provider rather than doctor. APRNs practicing at a state psychiatric facility, for example, may need to advocate for changes in or exceptions to the state drug formulary that prevents them from providing a specific antipsychotic medication proven effective for a specific patient.

Community-level advocacy is clearly needed to change small but significant perpetuation of APRN invisibility. For example, most automated messages used by pharmacies refer to doctors or doctors' representatives and need to be replaced by inclusive language of prescribers or providers. This situation provides important opportunities for reminding pharmacy management and business owners about the widespread contribution of APRN prescribers.

APRNs who educate their colleagues and supervisors about their legal scope of practice can advocate for the elimination of prescribing barriers that arise at a facility or in a practice. Facility or practice-level APRN councils, even when a small number of APRNs are involved, can lend credibility to advocacy efforts. Individuals are urged to assure that collaborative agreements do not include requirements beyond what the law stipulates.

Developing political competence for effective advocacy

APRNs will be most successful in their efforts to achieve fully autonomous prescribing when they achieve political competence in their interprofessional interactions. It is critical for APRNs to maintain their integrity and professional approach while being passionate but considered as they advocate for change. When APRNs develop consensus and cohesion, they promote an environment in which they are respected, trusted, and effective. O'Grady and Johnson (2009) eloquently articulate this perspective in their discourse on "Using force versus power" (see Box 3.5).

Box 3.5 Barriers to political competence

Using force versus power
Power accomplishes with ease what force, even with extreme effort, cannot. On the interpersonal front, it is important for APRNs to avoid using force in advancing their positions in the policy arena. This is commonly done by nurses participating in inter-disciplinary policy or problem-solving meetings. The twin approaches of being judgmental and parochial can quickly compromise effectiveness. *Judgmentalism[sic]*, or criticizing other people or disciplines, distracts from effective problem solving and in the process can reflect poorly on the judger, taking away the power to influence. When we diminish others or the work they do, we can provoke defensiveness and consequently limit ourselves and our capacity to influence others meaningfully. *Nursing parochialism* occurs when nurses present a narrow, restricted scope or outlook in which only nursing and nursing's interests are offered as solutions. These postures in the policy arena (or any other setting) do not build wide-based support or strong relationships. APRNs' potential impact on cost, quality, and access, if fully unleashed, is a powerful solution to some of the most perennial healthcare problems of our time. Power is characterized by humility and truth, which needs no defense or rhetoric – it is self-evident. Force is divisive and exploits people for individual or personal gain (Hawkins, 2002). For APRNs to be effective in influencing policy, a great degree of maturity, discipline, restraint, and respect for self and others must be practiced.

Source: O'Grady and Johnson (2009).

Box 3.6 Recommendation: prepare APRNs for a new scope of practice before legislation actually passes

Readiness for change could be enhanced by efforts to transition APRNs to a new scope of practice prior to the passage of legislation. Possible strategies to transition APRNs to a new scope of practice include the following:

- Develop a plan to prepare APRNs for scope of practice changes.
- Include formal and informal discussions at APRN conferences and meetings.
- Send informational mailings about the rationale for pending legislation to all APRNs licensed within a state (may require special funding).
- Encourage healthcare organizations that employ large numbers of APRNs to disseminate information using their internal communication mechanisms.
- Work with the media to communicate ongoing legislative activities.
- Work with legislators to include APRN legislative activities in their newsletters.
- Develop a collaborative project among all APRN groups and professional organizations within the state to establish a website dedicated to the implications of impending legislation.

Learning practical skills to influence policy positions the APRN to be effective in a variety of professional arenas. Many APRNs already have these skills honed from their professional experience and/or develop them further during graduate education. To enhance expertise, APRNs can attend educational offerings focused on policy. A mentor or experienced colleague can guide novices in the policy process. Volunteering for a professional organization's legislative or political action committee is an opportunity to gain direct experience and develop skills.

APRNs need to be prepared for changes in scope of practice. Education and outreach that informs APRNs, policymakers, and other health professionals of impending changes can facilitate adoption of new laws and regulations. Box 3.6 identifies a variety of strategies that can be used.

ELIMINATING INTERNAL BARRIERS TO PRESCRIBING

As APRNs engage in activities to eliminate external barriers and pass legislation that enables fully autonomous prescribing, attention to the elimination of internal barriers is equally as important. Moreover, efforts to prevent internal prescribing barriers need to begin in APRN educational programs. When internal barriers develop, they are often unacknowledged and can be more difficult to address than external barriers.

Role development in APRN programs

One component of APRN education is facilitating the transition of students from the role of administering medication to the role of prescribing medication. Course content and its application in clinical situations serve as the foundation for the prescriber role. APRN students develop prescribing competencies and expertise relevant to their scope of practice.

Some APRN educational programs are located in states that restrict APRN prescribing, particularly for CSs. Nonetheless, APRN programs are responsible for unambiguous socialization of students to assume the responsibilities of prescribing, including CSs. This is critical because complete prescriptive authority is an essential component of full practice authority. It is also important to prepare future APRNs in these states for scope of practice changes which may result from a change in the law or when moving to another state. APRN prescribing education that is consistent across states enhances professional mobility and prepares APRNs to practice in any state.

Professional development for the experienced APRN

APRNs who prescribe in restrictive environments are prone to developing internal barriers because they lack opportunities to utilize a full range of prescribing competencies. People tend to adapt to these environments and become less aware of their impact. Continuing education, conferences, journals, professional associations, and mentors are mechanisms to enhance awareness of these restrictions and encourage APRNs to overcome internal barriers.

Continuing education (CE) sessions typically update knowledge and prescribing competencies. CE can also address internal barriers and develop skills needed to deal with difficult situations, such as unwarranted requests for CSs. Professional conferences and meetings can serve as forums for APRNs to discuss internal barriers to prescribing and develop strategies to overcome them. Professional journals provide evidence-based prescribing information that supports continuous professional development.

IMPLICATIONS

External and internal prescribing barriers limit the ability of APRNs to reach their full professional potential. APRNs who practice in restrictive environments may underestimate the benefits of full practice authority. Faculty, preceptors, leaders, and individual APRNs share the responsibility to promote a vision of full practice authority as a right and responsibility. It is critical that students, who are the profession's future, internalize a keen understanding of the importance of autonomy for both their practice and profession. Each APRN's worldview makes a difference in building our collective strength to achieve full practice authority.

REFERENCES

Alabama Board of Nursing. (2019). Certified registered nurse practitioners, certified nurse midwife controlled drug certificate protocol. Retrieved from https://www.abn.alabama.gov/wp-content/uploads/2016/02/crnp-cnm-controlled-drug-protocol.pdf. (Accessed 7 September 2020.)

Andrilla, C.H.A., Jones, K.C., & Patterson, D.G. (2019). Prescribing practices of nurse practitioners and physician assistants waivered to prescribe buprenorphine and the barriers they experience prescribing buprenorphine. *Journal of Rural Health, 36*(2), 187–195.

Baker, D.W. (2017). The Joint Commission's pain standards: Origins and evolution. Retrieved from https://www.jointcommission.org/-/media/tjc/documents/

resources/pain-management/pain_std_history_web_version_05122017pdf. pdf?db=web&hash=e7d12a5c3be9df031f3d8fe0d8509580. (Accessed 7 September 2020.)

California Business and Professions Code. (2019). Chapter 6. Article 8. Section 2836. Retrieved from https://law.justia.com/codes/california/2019/code-bpc/division-2/chapter-6/article-8/section-2836-1/. (Accessed 7 September 2020.)

Code of Georgia. (2019). §43-34-25. Delegation of certain medical acts to advanced practice registered nurse; construction and limitations of such delegation; definitions; conditions of nurse protocol; issuance of prescription drug orders. Retrieved from https://law.justia.com/codes/georgia/2010/title-43/chapter-34/article-2/43-34-25. (Accessed 7 September 2020.)

Connecticut General Assembly. (2013). Chapter 420c* Controlled substance registration. Section 21a-317. Registration required. Retrieved from https://www.cga.ct.gov/current/pub/chap_420c.htm. (Accessed 7 September 2020.)

Drug Addiction Treatment Act of 2000. (2000). Public law 106-310-title. XXXV – Waiver authority for physicians who dispense or prescribe certain narcotic drugs for maintenance treatment or detoxification treatment. Retrieved fromhttps://www.govinfo.gov/content/pkg/plaw-106publ310/html/plaw-106publ310.htm. (Accessed 7 September 2020.)

Drug Enforcement Administration. (2006). Practitioner's manual: Section V valid prescription requirements. Retrieved from http://www.state.in.us/pla/files/dea_practitioner_manual.pdf. (Accessed 7 September 2020.)

Florida Administrative Code & Florida Administrative Register. (2017). Department of Health. Board of Medicine. Advanced registered nurse practitioners. Rule 64B8-35.002. Standards for Protocols. Retrieved from https://www.flrules.org/gateway/ruleno.asp?title=advanced%20registered%20nurse%20practitioner&id=64b8-35.002. (Accessed 7 September 2020.)

Georgia Comprehensive Rules & Regulations. (2019). Rule 410-11-14. Regulation of protocol. Use by advanced practice nurses as authorized by O.C.G.A. Section 43-34-26.3. Retrieved from http://rules.sos.ga.gov/gac/410-11-.14. (Accessed 7 September 2020.)

Hawkins, D. (2002). *Power vs. force: The hidden determinants of human behavior.* Alexandria, NSW: Hay House Publishing.

Kaplan, L., & Brown, M.A. (2008). Changing laws is not enough: Preparing ourselves for scope of practice changes. *American Journal for Nurse Practitioners, 12*(3), 52–53.

Kaplan, L., Brown, M.A., Andrilla, H., & Hart, L.G. (2006). Barriers to autonomous practice. *Nurse Practitioner, 31*(2), 57–63.

Kaplan, L., Brown, M.A., & Donahue, J. (2010). Prescribing controlled substances: How NPs in Washington are making a difference. *The Nurse Practitioner, 35*(5), 47–53.

Kentucky Administrative Regulations 20:059. (2013). 201 KAR 20:059. Advanced practice registered nurse controlled substances prescriptions. Retrieved from https://apps.legislature.ky.gov/law/kar/201/020/059.pdf. (Accessed 7 September 2020.)

Kentucky Revised Statutes. (2018). Chapter 314.011. Definitions for chapter "Advanced practice registered nursing." Retrieved from https://apps.legislature.ky.gov/law/statutes/statute.aspx?id=48246. (Accessed 7 September 2020.)

National Conference of State Legislatures. (2019). Prescribing policies: States confront opioid overdose epidemic. Retrieved from http://www.ncsl.org/research/health/prescribing-policies-states-confront-opioid-overdose-epidemic.aspx. (Accessed 7 September 2020.)

National Council of State Boards of Nursing. (2020). Member board profiles. Retrieved from https://www.ncsbn.org/profiles.htm. (Accessed 7 September 2020.)

Nebraska Revised Statute. (2017). Nebraska revised statute 28-414. Controlled substance; Schedule II; prescription; content. Retrieved from https://nebraskalegislature.gov/laws/statutes.php?statute=28-414. (Accessed 7 September 2020.)

O'Grady, E.T., & Johnson, J.E. (2009). Health policy issues in changing environments. In A.B. Hamric, J.A. Spross, & C.M. Hanson (Eds), *Advanced practice nursing: An integrative approach* (4th ed.). St. Louis, MO: Saunders Elsevier.

Pew Charitable Trusts. (2018). When are prescribers required to use prescription drug monitoring programs? Retrieved from https://www.pewtrusts.org/en/research-and-analysis/data-visualizations/2018/when-are-prescribers-required-to-use-prescription-drug-monitoring-programs. (Accessed 7 September 2020.)

Phillips, S.J. (2020). 32nd annual APRN legislative update. *The Nurse Practitioner,* 45(1), 28–55.

Public Health Service. (2018). Title 42. Chapter 1 Public Health Service. Department of Health and Human Services General Provisions. Part 8 Medication assisted treatment for opioid use disorder. Retrieved from https://www.govinfo.gov/content/pkg/cfr-2018-title42-vol1/pdf/cfr-2018-title42-vol1-part8.pdf. (Accessed 7 September 2020.)

Public Law 114-198. (2016). Comprehensive Addiction and Recovery Act. Retrieved from https://www.congress.gov/114/plaws/publ198/PLAW-114publ198.pdf. (Accessed 7 September 2020.)

Public Law 115-271. (2018). Substance Use-Disorder Prevention that Promotes Opioid Recovery and Treatment for Patients and Communities Act. Retrieved from https://www.congress.gov/115/plaws/publ271/PLAW-115publ271.pdf. (Accessed 7 September 2020.)

Public Law 116-136. (2020). Coronavirus Aid, Relief, and Economic Security Act. https://www.congress.gov/116/plaws/publ136/PLAW-116publ136.pdf. (Accessed 7 September 2020.)

Texas Administrative Code. (2013). Title 22 Examining boards. Part 9 Texas Medical Board. Chapter 193. Standing Delegation Orders. §193.7 Prescriptive authority agreements generally. Retrieved from http://txrules.elaws.us/rule/title22_chapter193. (Accessed 7 September 2020.)

Texas State Board of Pharmacy. (2019). Resources: Prescriptions which may be dispensed in Texas. Retrieved from https://www.pharmacy.texas.gov/files_pdf/quick_reference_guide.pdf. (Accessed 7 September 2020.)

Title 21 – Food and Drugs. (1970). 21 USC Chapter 13, subchapter I, Part B, 1970: Authority to control; standards and schedules. Retrieved from https://uscode.house.gov/view.xhtml?path=/prelim@title21/chapter13/subchapter1/partb&edition=prelim. (Accessed 7 September 2020.)

Utah Nurse Practice Act. (2013). Title 58. Chapter 31b-102 (13)(c) (iii). Retrieved from http://www.dopl.utah.gov/laws/58-31b.pdf. (Accessed 7 September 2020.)

Washington State Legislature. (n.d.). A citizen's guide to effective legislative participation. Retrieved from http://leg.wa.gov/legislature/pages/effectiveparticipation.aspx. (Accessed 7 September 2020.)

Regulation of Prescriptive Authority

4

Tracy Klein

This chapter provides an overview of the state and federal laws, regulations, and other factors that affect whether an advanced practice registered nurse (APRN) may prescribe autonomously. Fully autonomous prescribing is contrasted with examples of restricted prescribing authority. Discussion of the APRN Consensus Model highlights the opportunity for standardized regulation that achieves fully autonomous practice with full prescriptive authority and universal adoption of the term APRN.

Some states permit advanced practice registered nurses (APRNs) to independently assess, diagnose, and manage patients but restrict prescribing. As an example, APRNs might autonomously prescribe legend[1] drugs but require some type of physician involvement to prescribe controlled substances (Drug Enforcement Administration (DEA), 1993; National Council of State Boards of Nursing [NCSBN], 2020). All states, however, authorize nurse practitioners (NPs) to prescribe controlled substances (DEA, 1993), although some states limit the controlled substances an APRN may prescribe.

The majority of controlled substance restrictions pertain to Schedule II drugs which are the most controlled class of legally available drugs for patient use. Some states place other restrictions on prescribing controlled substances such as limiting the quantity that may be prescribed, or in the case of opioids the morphine equivalent dose (MED). An overview of the state and federal laws and regulations and other factors that affect whether an APRN may prescribe autonomously follows.

A MODEL FOR APRN FULL PRACTICE AUTHORITY

The *Consensus Model for APRN Regulation, Licensure, Accreditation, Certification and Education* (APRN Consensus Group & the National Council of State Boards of Nursing APRN Advisory Committee, 2008) is the first fully developed model of full practice authority for APRN practice intended for national adoption. The

---

[1] Legend drugs are any medications that require a prescription in the United States.

The Advanced Practice Registered Nurse as a Prescriber, Second Edition. Edited by Louise Kaplan and Marie Annette Brown.
© 2021 John Wiley & Sons Ltd. Published 2021 by John Wiley & Sons Ltd.

creation of this key document is indicative of the intent to change law, education, and recognition of APRNs to reflect practice to the full extent of licensure. This was a major accomplishment for the nursing profession and serves as a foundation to create a cohesive and uniform approach to advanced practice licensure, accreditation, certification, and education (LACE). APRN practice includes the clinical nurse specialist (CNS), certified nurse practitioner (CNP), certified nurse midwife (CNM), and certified registered nurse anesthetist (CRNA). The goal of the model is to promote recognition of full practice for APRNs by licensers, accreditors, certifiers, and educators. One of the Consensus Model's foundational requirements for boards of nursing is licensing APRNs as independent practitioners with no regulatory requirements for physician collaboration, direction, or supervision (APRN Consensus Group & the National Council of State Boards of Nursing APRN Advisory Committee, 2008). Based upon this definition, 22 states and the District of Columbia meet the definition of full practice authority. As an example, Box 4.1 is the section of Washington State's rules that identifies autonomous prescribing authority. Of note, states may still use various titles for an APRN (such as Washington's ARNP standing for Advanced Registered Nurse Practitioner), though uniformity is increasing in the United States.

Box 4.1 Washington law: autonomous prescribing

WAC [Washington Administrative Code] 246-840-400 ARNP prescriptive authority

(1) An ARNP licensed under chapter 18.79 RCW [Revised Code of Washington] when authorized by the nursing commission may prescribe drugs, medical equipment, and therapies pursuant to applicable state and federal laws.
(2) The ARNP, when exercising prescriptive authority, is accountable for competency in
(a) Problem identification through appropriate assessment;
(b) Medication or device selection;
(c) Patient education for use of therapeutics;
(d) Knowledge of interactions of therapeutics;
(e) Evaluation of outcome; and
(f) Recognition and management of side effects, adverse reactions and complications.

Source: From Washington Administrative Code 246-840-400, 2016. ARNP prescriptive authority. Public Domain.

Regulations for some APRN roles in various states may differ from those NPs who constitute the largest number of APRNs. Some states include CNMs as NPs, for example, while others license them as a separate role or through a separate regulatory board, which is the case in New York (New York State Education Department, 2019). NPs and CNMs have prescriptive authority in all 50 states and the District of Columbia. CNSs have no authority to prescribe in 16 states (NCSBN, 2020). Nurse anesthetists have no authority to prescribe in 16 states (NCSBN, 2020). When states restrict prescribing for the APRN, they often limit prescribing to a formulary or a narrow scope or may require a collaborative or supervisory relationship.

CONSENSUS MODEL FOR APRN REGULATION

LACE

The ability to autonomously prescribe legend drugs and controlled substances is still restricted for many APRNs despite an improved regulatory environment and the increased role of medications for therapeutic interventions with patients over more than a decade. LACE refers to the four elements of APRN regulation identified in the *Consensus Model for APRN Regulation* that are essential to implementation of the model. Each element plays a unique but interdependent role in how the APRN may exercise prescriptive authority. The legal ability to prescribe pharmacological and non-pharmacological interventions is one major differentiation between the APRN and registered nurse (RN) scopes of practice according to the LACE model (APRN Consensus & the National Council of State Boards of Nursing APRN Advisory Committee, 2008).

Licensing

The purpose of a regulatory licensing board is often misunderstood by the APRN. The primary purpose of a Board of Nursing is to protect the public. Licensing laws and requirements have been developed in the context of a libertarian theoretical perspective. This approach promotes government authority to the extent that core individual rights such as life, autonomy, and property are protected.

This context has three important implications for licensing laws. The first is the jurisdictional autonomy of each state's Board of Nursing to protect the public within that state. The second is the right of the state to determine and enforce its own laws and regulations as it sees fit (states' rights). The third is the right of the individual to legal protection against removal of private property. Both state and federal courts recognize a license as property that cannot be taken without due process (Hudspeth & Klein, 2019). Further, this protection is guaranteed under interpretation of the 14th Amendment and has been codified into state practice laws (Hudspeth & Klein, 2019).

All RNs are licensed through Boards of Nursing. In a few states, APRNs still practice under joint jurisdiction with Medical Boards (NCSBN, 2020). This model was commonly used in the 1970s when prescriptive authority was new. Authority by Medical Boards of APRNs was more often imposed in relation to prescribing than other aspects of practice.

APRNs in most, but not all, states require licensure as an RN and issuance of a second license. In August 1992, the NCSBN adopted a position paper advocating for a second license for APRN practice based upon the differences in scope of practice, including prescribing, from that of the RN (Edmunds, 1992; NCSBN, 1993). The need for a second license was opposed at that time by the American Nurses Association (ANA) based on the perspective that all nurses are under one scope of practice (Malone & Sheets, 1993). Since then, the evolution of advanced practice nursing and the accomplishments of APRNs have contributed to a deepened appreciation of APRN roles. The ANA, along with 40 other organizations, has endorsed the *Consensus Model for APRN Regulation*.

In some states, prescriptive authority is granted as part of APRN licensure, while in other states it is optional and requires a separate application. Prescribing authority may also require a separate designation or number, or registration with a Board of Medicine and/or Pharmacy. Michigan, while noted as a state with delegated prescriptive authority by the NCSBN (2020), passed legislation effective in 2017 which made delegated prescriptive authority applicable to controlled substances only (State of Michigan, 2016).

The ability to obtain prescriptive authority, whether restricted, optional, or mandatory, usually involves specific requirements (NCSBN, 2020). These include a minimum number of hours of pharmacology in the original educational program, pharmacotherapeutics continuing education (CE), collaborative agreements, and additional state prescribing licenses or DEA registration (NCSBN, 2020).

Some states do not permit autonomous or even collaborative prescriptive authority under the APRN's own license until completion of a supervised period of prescribing practice. Colorado requires a 1000-hour "mentorship" with a physician or advanced practice nurse with prescriptive authority; full prescriptive authority can then be authorized for NPs (Colorado Revised Statutes, 2019).

Accreditation

APRN programs are accredited by degree or role. Master's in Nursing and Doctor of Nursing Practice programs are accredited by the National League for Nursing Accreditation Commission (NLNAC), Accreditation Commission for Education in Nursing (ACEN), or Commission on Collegiate Nursing Education (CCNE). Nurse midwifery and nurse anesthetist programs are additionally accredited through the Accreditation Commission for Midwifery Education (ACME) and Council on Accreditation (COA) of Nurse Anesthesia programs, respectively.[2]

Standards and competencies for NPs developed by the National Organization of Nurse Practitioner Faculties (NONPF) are incorporated into the CCNE accreditation process of NP programs (National Task Force on Quality Nurse Practitioner Education, 2016). To ensure quality education, NONPF's core competencies for NP practice are used to develop curriculum and student outcomes. There is only one core competency related to prescribing.

APRN accreditation standards generally set criteria for pharmacology coursework. Educational programs determine how the course is applied in the curriculum and which components of state and federal prescribing laws to include. In addition to an advanced pharmacology course, pharmacological principles are integrated across the educational program and clinical practicals. The APRN student graduates with the ability to prescribe and manage patients using pharmacological therapy.

Certification

National certifying exams are developed by the professions to validate role, specialty, or population-specific competencies. APRN certification examinations validate entry-level knowledge and abilities for practice (Chornick, 2008). The

---

[2] APRN programs that are not in schools of nursing may only have ACME or COA accreditation.

majority of states require national certification for initial APRN licensure as well as maintenance of licensure (NCSBN, 2020). National certification has been required for CRNAs in order to qualify for Medicare reimbursement since 1992 (US Code of Federal Regulations, 2008). Subsequently, the Center for Medicare and Medicaid Services (CMS) required national certification for first-time NP, CNM, and CNS applicants (Centers for Medicare and Medicaid Services, 2001; US Code of Federal Regulations, 2013). Many state and private insurers also require national certification for credentialing.

National certification exams are based upon job analysis and role delineation studies that are updated periodically. At this time, the prescriber role, though integral to APRN practice, is a small component of national certification examinations. For example, pharmacological and prescribing content in the American Academy of Nurse Practitioners Certification Board (AANPCB) NP certification examination for family NPs includes questions related to pharmacology, pharmacotherapeutics management, and use of non-pharmacological or complementary therapies (AANPCB, 2019). National certification examinations do not test specifics of state law and requirements for prescribing. State-specific prescribing competencies should be included in the basic educational preparation for APRNs as well as incorporated into their ongoing licensure renewal requirements.

Education

Licensure, accreditation, and certification contribute to the educational design of curricula and preparation of APRNs as prescribers. Changes in practice are based on changing demographics, regional needs, patterns of migration, catastrophic events such as war, and evolution of APRN roles (Stievano et al., 2019). Even when state restrictions exist, all APRNs should be educated for autonomous practice to facilitate professional mobility.

NP and CRNA eligibility for national certification requires that the educational program verify completion of a minimum of three credits of graduate-level pharmacology. This requirement is consistent with the American Association of Colleges of Nursing's standards for doctoral and master's programs that prepare nurses for advanced practice. Educational programs should document through course descriptions, transcripts, and curricular materials the specific competencies necessary for prescriptive authority as they are developed throughout the curriculum and clinical practicals (Klein & Kaplan, 2010).

It is also the responsibility of educators to ensure that graduates are eligible for national certification and state licensure (APRN Consensus & the National Council of State Boards of Nursing APRN Advisory Committee, 2008). Distance learning programs and multiple campus delivery technology blur the boundaries of state-based education, increasing the responsibility of the student to carefully evaluate prescribing laws in the state where he or she will practice. Additionally, the ability to prescribe may not be available for a CRNA or a CNS in their chosen state of practice. This may create a need for additional education when the law changes to permit prescribing for the first time or when an APRN moves to another state and desires to apply for this authority (Klein & Kaplan, 2010).

There may be educational requirements, in addition to those in the initial program, when an APRN wants to reactivate licensure after a period of not practicing or prescribing. Reentry requirements for APRNs are developed on a state-by-state basis. Oregon, as an example, requires that an NP demonstrates at least 150 hours of utilizing pharmacological knowledge in order to renew licensure and prescriptive authority (Oregon Nurse Practice Act, 2019). Failure to do so requires completion of a 45-hour pharmacology course (Oregon Nurse Practice Act, 2019) and may also require an additional prescribing practicum.

Prescriptive authority renewal requirements for prescribing in some states may be met through CE courses. These may be offered by academic institutions, non-profit organizations, or for-profit CE companies. It is important to verify directly with the licensing board and national certifying organization which courses may be used toward renewal requirements. Boards and national certifying bodies generally accept nursing, pharmacy, or medical accreditation for pharmacology and prescribing courses. Common accrediting bodies include the Accreditation Council for Pharmacy Education, the Accreditation Council for Medical Education, and the American Nurses Credentialing Center.

HISTORY OF APRN PRESCRIBING REGULATION

Idaho was the first state to pass a law authorizing prescriptive authority for NPs in 1971 (R. Hudspeth, personal communication, December 27, 2009). The law was not implemented until 1977 due to protracted requirements for joint rulemaking with the Board of Medicine (S. Evans, personal communication, December 28, 2009). Other states also authorized APRN prescriptive authority in the 1970s: Washington, Oregon, New Mexico, Florida (CRNAs), North Carolina, Utah, and Maryland (CRNAs). CNSs were often granted prescriptive authority if they specialized in psychiatry. The number of states granting prescriptive authority increased rapidly during the 1980s and 1990s (Hamric et al., 2009). However, as late as 1983, only Oregon and Washington State granted NPs and CNMs statutory autonomous prescriptive authority. Oregon's authority included Schedule III–V controlled substances. Washington's law included only Schedule V controlled substances but also extended to CRNAs.

In order to prescribe controlled substances, APRNs must register with the DEA and some states may also require additional registration with a Board of Pharmacy. Not until 1993 did the DEA adopt the category "Mid-Level Provider" which permitted APRNs to register under their own unique name and number and mandated that they do so if they were prescribing controlled substances (DEA, 1993). Before 1993, registration of APRNs was done on a case-by-case basis in states that had existing autonomous prescribing authority (C. Brennan, personal communication, January 14, 2010).

During the late 1980s, CRNAs sought clarification as to whether prescribing was part of their practice. The DEA concluded that CRNAs administer medications and anesthetics in the perianesthesia period and this is considered administration or dispensing, but not prescribing (Blumenreich, 1988). APRNs who administer and dispense controlled substances as the agent of a person or facility registered with the DEA are exempt from individual registration (Blumenreich, 1993; DEA, 1993). These issues are particularly relevant to

CRNAs who administer or dispense controlled substances routinely without prescriptive authority or an individual DEA registration (Blumenreich, 1993; Kaplan et al., 2011), though a majority of states now include prescriptive authority for CRNAs under their own license.

Between 2001 and 2010 the general trends in regulating prescriptive authority included raising educational requirements, decreasing requirements for physician involvement, and increasing the schedule of controlled substance that can be prescribed by APRNs (Gadbois et al., 2015). Guidelines to restrict prescribing opioids were initiated by Washington state in 2011, and passage by multiple states followed based on the increase in opioid deaths and misuse across the United States (Davis, n.d.). Since that time, numerous states have passed laws limiting both dose and quantity of opioids that may be prescribed (National Conference of State Legislatures, 2019). Ironically, state law also sometimes constrains NPs from prescribing medication assisted therapies which may alleviate opioid use disorder (Jackson & Lopez, 2018).

AUTONOMOUS PRESCRIPTIVE AUTHORITY

Autonomous prescribing is the ability to legally and independently select, prescribe, administer, dispense, and manage pharmacological treatments for individual patients regardless of setting, time frame, or circumstance. Having full practice authority in a state does not mean a state or employer cannot still limit prescribing functions. Practice barriers that focus on prescribing may restrict autonomous prescribing significantly. Examples of restrictions related to APRN prescribing include:

- Requirements for a significant period of physician supervised practice before autonomous prescriptive authority is granted
- Joint jurisdiction with a medical or pharmacy board which determines scope and function of prescriptive authority or practice
- Requirements to prescribe under a physician's supervision
- Site-based authority
- Formularies that designate in state law what type or quantity of drug may be prescribed

Box 4.2 shows a section of the Virginia law that requires joint jurisdiction of APRNs by the Board of Nursing and Board of Medicine. This constrains all APRNs to joint regulation with allowance for NPs only to obtain a degree of practice autonomy after a period of supervised practice (five years in this case).

Box 4.2 Virginia law: joint jurisdiction

§ 54.1-2957. Licensure of nurse practitioners (Code of Virginia, 2019)

B. The Board of Medicine and the Board of Nursing shall jointly prescribe the regulations governing the licensure of nurse practitioners. It shall be unlawful for a person to practice as a nurse practitioner in this Commonwealth unless he holds such a joint license.

(Continued)

I. A nurse practitioner, other than a nurse practitioner licensed by the Boards of Medicine and Nursing in the category of certified nurse midwife or certified registered nurse anesthetist, who has completed the equivalent of at least five years of full-time clinical experience as a licensed nurse practitioner, as determined by the Boards, may practice in the practice category in which he is certified and licensed without a written or electronic practice agreement upon receipt by the nurse practitioner of an attestation from the patient care team physician stating (i) that the patient care team physician has served as a patient care team physician on a patient care team with the nurse practitioner pursuant to a practice agreement meeting the requirements of this section and § 54.1-2957.01; (ii) that while a party to such practice agreement, the patient care team physician routinely practiced with a patient population and in a practice area included within the category for which the nurse practitioner was certified and licensed; and (iii) the period of time for which the patient care team physician practiced with the nurse practitioner under such a practice agreement. A copy of such attestation shall be submitted to the Boards together with a fee established by the Boards. Upon receipt of such attestation and verification that a nurse practitioner satisfies the requirements of this subsection, the Boards shall issue to the nurse practitioner a new license that includes a designation indicating that the nurse practitioner is authorized to practice without a practice agreement. In the event that a nurse practitioner is unable to obtain the attestation required by this subsection, the Boards may accept other evidence demonstrating that the applicant has met the requirements of this subsection in accordance with regulations adopted by the Boards. A nurse practitioner authorized to practice without a practice agreement pursuant to this subsection shall (a) only practice within the scope of his clinical and professional training and limits of his knowledge and experience and consistent with the applicable standards of care, (b) consult and collaborate with other health care providers based on the clinical conditions of the patient to whom health care is provided, and (c) establish a plan for referral of complex medical cases and emergencies to physicians or other appropriate health care providers.

APRNs may perceive that they have autonomous prescriptive authority despite the presence of significant legal or regulatory barriers. This is sometimes true of APRNs who prescribe in states that require a collaborative or supervisory agreement with a physician only when prescribing controlled substances. These APRNs may create a practice without controlled substances or normalize this limitation and describe themselves as an autonomous prescriber. However, changes in the practice environment such as a new job can prompt them to recognize the limits that the law imposes (Kaplan et al., 2006). Some APRNs practice without taking advantage of the legal option for autonomous prescriptive authority. Perceived barriers such as the cost of DEA registration, liability, or discomfort in changing the status quo can contribute to self-imposed limitations in prescribing (Craig-Rodriguez et al., 2017; Kaplan & Brown, 2007).

Collaboration
Interprofessional collaboration need not be a barrier to autonomous prescribing and is an important aspect of comprehensive patient care (Institute of

Medicine [IOM], 2003). Collaborative care provided within interdisciplinary teams should be a professional norm for all health professionals in practice (IOM, 2003). In contrast, mandatory collaboration by regulatory restriction of licensed, credentialed APRNs is widespread, and its elimination is the goal of the APRN Consensus Model. The implementation and structure of collaborative agreements vary widely from state to state. Lack of mandated collaborative agreements has been linked to improved patient outcomes and healthcare utilization (Traczynski & Udalova, 2018; Xue et al., 2016).

In an ideal pluralistic environment, healthcare professionals would share political and economic power. Instead, organized medicine through groups such as the American Medical Association (AMA) has consistently used the legislative and regulatory processes to oppose autonomous prescribing by APRNs and exert financial and political pressure to restrict expansion of scope of practice. It is the position of the AMA (1999, 2009, 2016) that NPs, as well as all other categories of prescribers other than physicians, should not be permitted to autonomously practice. The AMA also provides funding to monitor and oppose legislation which would grant autonomous prescribing.

Lugo et al. (2007) identified factors that impact the ability of NPs to provide care and highlighted how the regulatory environment affects patient access to prescription medications. Restrictive prescribing laws result in an underrepresentation of the number and type of prescriptions generated by APRNs. In states with restrictions, prescriptions are often tracked under the supervising or collaborating physician's name or DEA number. Autonomous prescribing by all APRNs is necessary to accurately determine characteristics of APRN prescribing. The advent of prescription drug monitoring programs (PDMPS) to evaluate controlled substance prescribing may offer further opportunities to evaluate and link patient outcomes to prescribing practices. PDMPs are now active in all 50 states (Prescription Drug Monitoring Program Training and Technical Assistance Center, 2020).

The National Provider Identifier

The National Plan and Provider Enumeration System includes a unique 10-digit registration for healthcare providers known as the National Provider Identifier (NPI) (US Centers for Medicare and Medicaid Services, 2020). Prior to inception of the NPI, pharmacies often required a DEA number from prescribers for tracking purposes even if a controlled substance was not being prescribed. The NPI serves as a billing identifier for most healthcare providers regardless of their regulatory status. You must have an NPI in order to enroll in Medicare as a provider, and an NPI is required to bill for items that may be authorized through use of a prescription such as Durable Medical Equipment (Department of Health and Human Services, 2016). The NPI number could potentially be used to more accurately track APRN prescribing, which could be of great benefit by demonstrating the role APRNs play in prescribing.

OTHER REGULATORY REQUIREMENTS

APRNs may be credentialed by healthcare systems as licensed independent practitioners under the Joint Commission guidelines adopted in their ambulatory care manual (Joint Commission on Accreditation of Healthcare Organizations, 2020). In states where autonomous practice is legally permitted, facilities may credential an APRN to admit, discharge, manage, and prescribe for patients on an inpatient or outpatient basis. There is limited legal or regulatory guidance regarding credentialing to practice within a facility (Klein, 2008). When credentialing, a facility may limit prescribing or restrict an APRN's legal scope of practice but may not broaden it beyond state and federal law.

Federal agencies such as the Veterans Health Administration (VA) may also credential an APRN to prescribe. These agencies require the APRN to have state licensure (not necessarily in the state of practice) and credentialing within the VA (US Department of Veterans Affairs, 2018). As of 2017, APRNs who are CNSs, CNMs, or NPs (but not CRNAs) may be recognized within the VA as having full practice authority regardless of their state of licensure requirements (US Department of Veterans Affairs, 2017).

PRESCRIPTIVE AUTHORITY LIMITATIONS

There are many types of limitation to prescriptive authority, not all of which are legally imposed. It is important for APRNs to understand the source of a prescribing limit in order to effect change. Limits to prescribing for APRNs may originate in law, regulation, policy, or custom. Some limits to prescribing apply specifically to controlled substances and apply to all prescribers, not just APRNs (see Box 4.3).

Box 4.3 Utah Controlled Substances Act Rules (2019): applies to all prescribers

R156-37-603. Restrictions upon the prescription, dispensing and administration of controlled substances

(1) A practitioner may prescribe or administer the Schedule II controlled substance cocaine hydrochloride only as a topical anesthetic for mucous membranes in surgical situations in which it is properly indicated and as local anesthetic for the repair of facial and pediatric lacerations when the controlled substance is mixed and dispensed by a registered pharmacist in the proper formulation and dosage.
(2) A practitioner shall not prescribe or administer a controlled substance without taking into account the drug's potential for abuse, the possibility the drug may lead to dependence, the possibility the patient will obtain the drug for a non-therapeutic use or to distribute to others, and the possibility of an illicit market for the drug.
(3) When writing a prescription for a controlled substance, each prescription shall contain only one controlled substance per prescription form and no other legend drug or prescription item shall be included on that form.

---

(4) In accordance with Subsection 58-37-6(7)(f)(v)(D), unless the prescriber determines there is a valid medical reason to allow an earlier dispensing date, the dispensing date of a second or third prescription shall be no less than 30 days from the dispensing date of the previous prescription, to allow for receipt of the subsequent prescription before the previous prescription runs out.

(5) If a practitioner fails to document his intentions relative to refills of controlled substances in Schedules III through V on a prescription form, it shall mean no refills are authorized. No refill is permitted on a prescription for a Schedule II controlled substance.

(6) Refills of controlled substance prescriptions shall be permitted for the period from the original date of the prescription as follows: (a) Schedules III and IV for 6 months from the original date of the prescription; and (b) Schedule V for 1 year from the original date of the prescription.

(7) No refill may be dispensed until such time has passed since the date of the last dispensing that 80% of the medication in the previous dispensing should have been consumed if taken according to the prescriber's instruction.

(8) No prescription for a controlled substance shall be issued or dispensed without specific instructions from the prescriber on how and when the drug is to be used.

(9) Refills after expiration of the original prescription term requires the issuance of a new prescription by the prescribing practitioner.

(10) Each prescription for a controlled substance and the number of refills authorized shall be documented in the patient records by the prescribing practitioner.

(11) A practitioner shall not prescribe or administer a Schedule II controlled stimulant for any purpose except
  (a) the treatment of narcolepsy as confirmed by neurological evaluation;
  (b) the treatment of abnormal behavioral syndrome, attention deficit disorder, hyperkinetic syndrome, or related disorders;
  (c) the treatment of drug-induced brain dysfunction;
  (d) the differential diagnostic psychiatric evaluation of depression;
  (e) the treatment of depression shown to be refractory to other therapeutic modalities, including pharmacological approaches, such as tricyclic antidepressants or MAO inhibitors;
  (f) in the terminal stages of disease, as adjunctive therapy in the treatment of chronic severe pain or chronic severe pain accompanied by depression;
  (g) the clinical investigation of the effects of the drugs, in which case the practitioner shall submit to the division a written investigative protocol for its review and approval before the investigation has begun. The investigation shall be conducted in strict compliance with the investigative protocol, and the practitioner shall, within 60 days following the conclusion of the investigation, submit to the division a written report detailing the findings and conclusions of the investigation; or
  (h) in treatment of depression associated with medical illness after due consideration of other therapeutic modalities.

Some prescribing limits have their foundation in safety, efficacy, cost, availability, or patient-specific indications. For example, an insurer may limit coverage of a medication to its standardized dosing parameters for the average individual patient or limit the number of pills that are a covered benefit each month. The Food and Drug Administration may require that a drug such as Accutane be prescribed as part of a "limited access program" to specific patient populations such as people for whom more than one birth control method has been confirmed due to significant fetal risk. Other limits are not in alignment with current practice and law, such as the restriction on providing buprenorphine for opioid addiction, which is legal federally, by states that do not allow NPs to prescribe it (Spetz et al., 2019). The safe prescriber self-evaluates to identify limits to prescribing in accordance with scope of practice, knowledge, competency, and evidence. A discussion of specific strategies to address and remove prescribing limitations can be found in Chapter 3.

Medication samples

Many nurse practice acts specifically include language regarding the APRNs' ability to receive, distribute, and sign for samples as part of their prescriptive authority. The Prescription Drug Marketing Act (PDMA) of 1987 was intended to address drug diversion and sales of samples by providing regulations to track their distribution (Angarola & Beach, 1996; Food and Drug Administration, 2009; Romanski, 2003). Implementation of the law in 2000, however, resulted in many APRNs being denied the ability to sign for or receive samples without a supervising physician signature. There was confusion about prescribing requirements among drug companies which found it difficult to review and evaluate APRN prescribing laws state by state. Currently, dispensing of medication samples has been curtailed in many offices over concerns regarding drug storage and interruption of clinical flow. Sample use and distribution in the United States has decreased overall as generics replace commonly sampled drugs (Brown et al., 2017). Medical marketing in the United States now focuses primarily on direct to patient marketing, direct payment to prescribers (primarily physicians), and disease education (Schwartz & Woloshin, 2019).

Formularies

Some Boards of Nursing, when required by law, adopted formularies for APRN prescribing. A formulary is a list of drugs, drug classes, or drug categories that may be prescribed by health professionals within the scope of their licensure. Many formularies required approval by physicians and/or pharmacists, in conjunction with input from nurse prescribers. States such as Oregon and New Hampshire adopted formularies as a compromise to enable other aspects of autonomous practice (Pruitt et al., 2002). Once adopted, formularies can take many years to remove. Oregon's formulary requirement was removed in 2008 after 29 years (State of Oregon, 2008), while the New Hampshire formulary requirement was removed in 2009 after 25 years (Sampson, 2009; State of New Hampshire, 2009). Restriction to prescribing from a formulary is much less common than when APRNs were initially regulated and currently only 2-4% of states use a formulary depending on APRN role (NCSBN, 2020).

Dispensing

The DEA (2016) defines dispensing as follows:

> The term "dispense" means to deliver a controlled substance to an ultimate user or research subject by, or pursuant to the lawful order of, a practitioner, including the prescribing and administering of a controlled substance and the packaging, labeling or compounding necessary to prepare the substance for such delivery. The term "dispenser" means a practitioner who so delivers a controlled substance to an ultimate user or research subject.

State law that defines dispensing may be more restrictive than the federal definition. Box 4.4 defines Oregon dispensing law for nurses with prescriptive authority. Broader dispensing authority is primarily accorded to physicians, pharmacists, and veterinarians. The ability to apply for and be granted dispensing authority varies greatly for APRNs from state to state. APRNs have been subject in state law to limitations on their dispensing authority as well as their ability to distribute samples. Examples of dispensing restrictions may include geographic location, ability to charge or bill, quantity, type of medication, and patient population.

Box 4.4 Oregon law: dispensing limits

678.390 Authority of nurse practitioner and clinical nurse specialist to write prescriptions or dispense drugs; notice; requirements; revocation; rules

(1) The Oregon State Board of Nursing authorize a licensed nurse practitioner or licensed clinical nurse specialist to write prescriptions including prescription for controlled substances listed in schedules II, III, IIIN, IV and V.

(2) A licensed nurse practitioner or licensed clinical nurse specialist may submit an application to the Oregon State Board of Nursing to dispense prescription drugs. The Oregon State Board of Nursing shall provide immediate notice to the State Board of Pharmacy upon approving an application from a licensed nurse practitioner or licensed clinical nurse specialist.

(3) An application for the authority to dispense prescription drugs under this section must include any information required by the Oregon State Board of Nursing by rule.

(4) Prescription drugs dispensed by a licensed nurse practitioner or licensed clinical nurse specialist must be personally dispensed by the licensed nurse practitioner or licensed clinical nurse specialist, except that nonjudgmental dispensing functions may be delegated to staff assistants when:

    (a) The accuracy and completeness of the prescription is verified by the licensed nurse practitioner or licensed clinical nurse specialist; and

    (b) The prescription drug is labeled with the name of the patient to whom it is being dispensed.

(5) The Oregon State Board of Nursing shall adopt rules requiring:

    (a) Prescription drugs dispensed by licensed nurse practitioners and licensed clinical nurse specialists to be either prepackaged by a manufacturer registered with the State Board of Pharmacy or repackaged by a pharmacist licensed by the State Board of Pharmacy under ORS chapter 689;

(Continued)

(b) Labeling requirements for prescription drugs dispensed by licensed nurse practitioners and licensed clinical nurse specialists that are the same as labeling requirements required of pharmacies licensed under ORS chapter 689;

(c) Record keeping requirements for prescriptions and prescription drug dispensing by a licensed nurse practitioner and a licensed clinical nurse specialist that are the same as the record keeping requirements required of pharmacies licensed under ORS chapter 689;

(d) A dispensing licensed nurse practitioner and a dispensing licensed clinical nurse specialist to have available at the dispensing site a hard copy or electronic version of prescription drug reference works commonly used by professionals authorized to dispense prescription medications; and

(e) A dispensing licensed nurse practitioner and a dispensing licensed clinical nurse specialist to allow representatives of the State Board of Pharmacy, upon receipt of a complaint, to inspect a dispensing site after prior notice to the Oregon State Board of Nursing.

(6) The Oregon State Board of Nursing has sole disciplinary authority regarding licensed nurse practitioners and licensed clinical nurse specialists who have prescription drug dispensing authority.

(7) The authority to write prescriptions or dispense prescription drugs may be denied, suspended or revoked by the Oregon State Board of Nursing upon proof that the authority has been abused. The procedure shall be a contested case under ORS chapter 183. Disciplinary action under this subsection is grounds for discipline of the licensed nurse practitioner or licensed clinical nurse specialist in the same manner as a licensee may be disciplined under ORS 678.111.

APRNs who dispense medications may be required to obtain a separate dispensing license and meet specific criteria. Alternatively, dispensing authority may be included as part of prescriptive authority. In addition, some states mandate dispensing limits for controlled substances. Kentucky, Alabama, Arizona, Nebraska, and many other states completely prohibit dispensing of controlled substances by NPs (DEA, 1993).

Quantity limitations

The quantity of medications prescribed or dispensed by APRNs is sometimes limited by state law. A search of the literature revealed no evidence that a restriction in the amount of typical medication prescribed or dispensed by APRNs is necessary to assure APRNs offer quality care. However, increasingly, opioids are limited in law for all types of prescribers, due to Centers for Disease Control and Prevention guidance on appropriate management of chronic pain and increased awareness of the opioid crisis and its impact (Dowell et al., 2016). Such limits may be expressed as quantity or morphine equivalent dose (MED) per day. In 2018, Senate bill 2456, known as CARA 2.0 Act, was introduced, proposing that federal law limit any prescribing of opioids for acute pain to a three-day supply (CARA 2.0 Act, 2018). Although this legislation did not pass, there is an increasing call to address the inappropriate prescribing of controlled substances in state and federal law.

Co-signatures

States with supervision or collaborative agreements do not require a physician to co-sign prescriptions. An APRN with prescriptive authority for a class of drugs may sign the prescription unless the collaborative agreement stipulates that the physician must also sign. An example of this type of clarification can be found in New York, which provides explicit detail regarding the requirements of collaborative agreements (New York State Education Department, 2015).

Mail order/prescribing across state lines

The ability to fill a prescription written by an APRN from another state is either specifically permitted or at the pharmacist's discretion in accordance with state pharmacy law. It is increasingly more common for insurers to encourage use of mail-order pharmacies, often located outside the APRN's state, causing confusion regarding APRN prescribing authority. The adoption of uniform and consistent requirements for APRN prescribing would reduce this type of confusion.

CONCLUSION

APRN authority to prescribe varies greatly from state-to-state and among APRN roles. Disparities among national APRN regulations related to prescribing reflect diverse sociocultural and political norms and may affect the professional development of the APRN prescriber. National adoption in law of the APRN Consensus Model is helping to eliminate these disparities. Evidence-based prescribing competencies can also be used to develop uniform regulatory requirements. The ultimate goal is to create the opportunity for APRNs to practice to the full scope of their expertise and to establish autonomous and responsible prescribing authority for all APRNs (Klein & Kaplan, 2010).

REFERENCES

American Academy of Nurse Practitioners Certification Board. (2019). FNP examination blueprint. Retrieved from https://www.aanpcert.org/certs/fnp. (Accessed 7 September 2020.)

American Medical Association. (1999). Report of the Council on Medical Service. Non-physician prescribing. Resolution 511, A-98. Chicago: American Medical Association.

American Medical Association. (2009). *AMA scope of practice data series: Nurse practitioners*. Chicago: American Medical Association.

American Medical Association (2016). AMA statement on VA proposed rules on advanced practice nurses. Chicago: American Medical Association.

Angarola, R., & Beach, J. (1996). The Prescription Drug Marketing Act: A solution in search of a problem? *Food and Drug Law Journal, 51*(1), 21–55.

APRN Consensus Group & the National Council of State Boards of Nursing APRN Advisory Committee. (2008). Consensus Model for APRN Regulation, Licensure, Accreditation, Certification & Education. Chicago: NCSBN.

Blumenreich, G.A. (1988). Nurse anesthetists and prescriptive authority. *Journal of the American Association of Nurse Anesthetists, 56*(2), 91–93.

Blumenreich, G.A. (1993). Legal briefs: Drug Enforcement Administration Mid-level Practitioner Regulation. Retrieved from https://www.aana.com/docs/default-source/aana-journal-web-documents-1/legal_briefs_1093_p480.pdf?sfvrsn=323655b1_4.

Brown, J.D., Doshi, P.A., & Talbert, J.C. (2017). Utilization of free medication samples in the United States in a nationally representative sample: 2009–2013. *Research in Social & Administrative Pharmacy, 13*(1), 193–200.

CARA 2.0 Act. (2018). S.2456 – 115th Congress (2017–2018). Retrieved from https://www.congress.gov/bill/115th-congress/senate-bill/2456/text. (Accessed 7 September 2020.)

Centers for Medicare and Medicaid Services. (2001). Medicare carriers manual Part 3 – claims process: Transmittal 1734. Retrieved from https://www.cms.gov/regulations-and-guidance/guidance/transmittals/downloads/r1734b3.pdf. (Accessed 7 September 2020.)

Chornick, N. (2008). APRN licensure versus APRN certification: what is the difference? *JONAS Healthcare Law Ethics and Regulation, 10*(4), 90–93.

Code of Virginia. (2019). §54.1 – 2957. Licensure and practice of nurse practitioners. Retrieved from https://law.lis.virginia.gov/vacode/title54.1/chapter29/section54.1-2957/. (Accessed 7 September 2020.)

Colorado Revised Statutes. (2019). Title 12, Article 255 Nurses. Retrieved from https://www.colorado.gov/pacific/dora/nursing_laws. (Accessed 7 September 2020.)

Craig-Rodriguez, A., Gordon, G., Kaplan, L., & Grubbs, L. (2017). Transitioning Florida NPs to opioid prescribing. *The Nurse Practitioner, 42*(9), 1–8.

Davis, C. (n.d.). State by state summary of opioid prescribing regulations and guidelines. Retrieved from https://www.azdhs.gov/documents/prevention/womens-childrens-health/injury-prevention/opioid-prevention/appendix-b-state-by-state-summary.pdf. (Accessed 7 September 2020.)

Department of Health and Human Services. (2016). NPI: What you need to know. Retrieved from https://www.cms.gov/outreach-and-education/medicare-learning-network-mln/mlnproducts/downloads/npi-what-you-need-to-know.pdf. (Accessed 7 September 2020.)

Dowell, D., Haegerich, T.M., & Chou, R. (2016). CDC guideline for prescribing opioids for chronic pain – United States. *Morbidity and Mortality Weekly Report (MMWR), 65*(21), 1–49.

Drug Enforcement Administration. (1993). Definition and registration of mid-level practitioners. Federal Register, Vol. *58*, No. 107. Retrieved from https://www.deadiversion.usdoj.gov/fed_regs/rules/prior_1998/fr0607_1993.htm. (Accessed 7 September 2020.)

Drug Enforcement Administration. (2016). Title 21 United States Code (USC) Controlled Substances Act. Section 802. Definitions. Retrieved from https://www.deadiversion.usdoj.gov/21cfr/21usc/802.htm. (Accessed 7 September 2020.)

Drug Enforcement Administration. (2019). Mid-level practitioners authorization by state. Retrieved from https://www.deadiversion.usdoj.gov/drugreg/practioners/mlp_by_state.pdf. (Accessed 7 September 2020.)

Edmunds, M. (1992). Council's pursuit of national standardization for advanced practice nursing meets with resistance. *The Nurse Practitioner, 17*(10), 81–83.

Food and Drug Administration. (2009). Prescription Drug Marketing Act of 1987. Retrieved from https://www.fda.gov/regulatory-information/selected-amendments-fdc-act/prescription-drug-marketing-act-1987. (Accessed 7 September 2020.)

Gadbois, E.A., Miller, E.A., Tyler, D., & Intrator, O. (2015). Trends in state regulation of nurse practitioners and physician assistants, 2001 to 2010. *Medical Care Research and Review, 72*(2), 200–219.

Hamric, A.B., Spross, J.A., & Hanson, C.M. (Eds). (2009). *Advanced practice nursing: An integrative approach* (4th ed.). St. Louis, MO: Elsevier.

Hudspeth, R.S., & Klein, T.A. (2019). Understanding nurse practitioner scope of practice: Regulatory, practice, and employment perspectives now and for the future. *Journal of the American Association of Nurse Practitioners, 31*(8), 468–473.

Institute of Medicine. (2003). *Health professions education: A bridge to quality.* Washington, DC: National Academies Press.

Jackson, H.J., & Lopez, C.M. (2018). Utilization of the nurse practitioner role to combat the opioid crisis. *Journal for Nurse Practitioners, 14*(10), e213–e216.

Joint Commission on Accreditation of Healthcare Organizations. (2020). *2020 Accreditation standards.* Oakbrook Terrace, IL: Joint Commission on Accreditation of Healthcare Organizations.

Kaplan, L., & Brown, M.A. (2007). The transition of nurse practitioners to changes in prescriptive authority. *Journal of Nursing Scholarship, 39*(2), 184–190.

Kaplan, L., Brown, M.A., Andrilla, H., & Hart, L.G. (2006). Barriers to autonomous practice. *Nurse Practitioner, 31*(1), 57–63.

Kaplan, L., Brown, M.A., & Simonson, D.C. (2011). CRNA prescribing practices: The Washington state experience. *AANA Journal, 79*(1), 24–29.

Klein, T. (2008). Credentialing the nurse practitioner in your workplace. *Nursing Administration Quarterly, 32*(4), 273–278.

Klein, T., & Kaplan, L. (2010). Prescribing competencies for advanced practice registered nurses. *Journal for Nurse Practitioners, 6*(2), 115–122.

Lugo, N., O'Grady, E., Hodnicki, D., & Hanson, C. (2007). Ranking state NP regulation: Practice environment and consumer health-care choice. *American Journal for Nurse Practitioners, 11*(4), 8–24.

Malone, B., & Sheets, V. (1993). Second licensure? ANA and NCSBN debate the issue. *The American Nurse, 25*(8), 8–9.

National Conference of State Legislatures. (2019). Prescribing policies: states confront opioid overdose epidemic. Retrieved from https://www.ncsl.org/research/health/prescribing-policies-states-confront-opioid-overdose-epidemic.aspx. (Accessed 7 September 2020.)

National Council of State Boards of Nursing. (1993). Regulation of advanced nursing practice: NCSBN position paper, 1993. Retrieved from https://www.ncsbn.org/737.htm. (Accessed 7 September 2020.)

National Council of State Boards of Nursing. (2020). Member board profiles. Retrieved from https://www.ncsbn.org/profiles.htm. (Accessed 7 September 2020.)

National Task Force on Quality Nurse Practitioner Education. (2016). *Criteria for evaluation of nurse practitioner programs.* Washington, DC: National Organization of Nurse Practitioner Faculties.

New York State Education Department. (2015). Practice requirements for nurse practitioners. Retrieved from http://www.op.nysed.gov/prof/nurse/np-prfnp.pdf. (Accessed 7 September 2020.)

New York State Education Department. (2019). License requirements. Retrieved from http://www.op.nysed.gov/prof/midwife/midwifelic.htm. (Accessed 7 September 2020.)

Oregon Nurse Practice Act. (2019). Division 56. Retrieved from https://www.oregon.gov/osbn/pages/laws-rules.aspx. (Accessed 7 September 2020.)

Prescription Drug Monitoring Program Training and Technical Assistance Center. (2020). State PDMP profiles and contacts. Retrieved from https://www.pdmpassist.org/content/state-pdmp-websites?order=field_state_territory_district_value&sort=asc. (Accessed 7 September 2020.)

Pruitt, R., Wetsel, M.A., Smith, K., & Spitler, H. (2002). How do we pass NP autonomy legislation? *The Nurse Practitioner, 27*(3), 56–65.

Romanski, J. (2003). The final sampling regulations of the Prescription Drug Monitoring Act are alive and well: Is your sampling program compliant? *Food and Drug Law Journal, 58*(4), 649–660.

Sampson, D. (2009). Alliances of cooperation: Negotiating New Hampshire nurse practitioners' prescribing practice. *Nursing History Review, 17*(1), 153–178.

Schwartz, L.M., & Woloshin, S. (2019). Medical marketing in the United States, 1997–2016. *JAMA, 321*(1), 80–96.

Spetz, J., Toretsky, C., & Chapman, S. (2019). Nurse practitioner and physician assistant waivers to prescribe buprenorphine and state scope of practice restrictions. *JAMA, 321*(14), 1407–1408.

State of Michigan. (2016). Enrolled House Bill No. 5400. Retrieved from https://www.legislature.mi.gov/documents/2015-2016/publicact/pdf/2016-pa-0499.pdf. (Accessed 7 September 2020.)

State of New Hampshire. (2009). New Hampshire Senate Bill 66. Chapter 54 Stat. Ann. Retrieved from https://legiscan.com/nh/text/sb66/id/1463691. (Accessed 7 September 2020.)

State of Oregon. (2008). SB 1062, ORS 678.375, Section 2, Stat. Ann. Retrieved from https://www.oregonlaws.org/ors/678.375. (Accessed 7 September 2020.)

Stievano, A., Caruso, R., Pittella, F., et al. (2019). Shaping nursing profession regulation through history – a systematic review. *International Nursing Review, 66*(1), 17–29.

Traczynski, J., & Udalova, V. (2018). Nurse practitioner independence, health care utilization, and health outcomes. *Journal of Health Economics, 58*, 90–109.

US Centers for Medicare and Medicaid Services. (2020). NPPES NPI registry. Retrieved from https://npiregistry.cms.hhs.gov/. (Accessed 7 September 2020.)

US Code of Federal Regulations. (2008). Services of a certified registered nurse anesthetist or an anesthesiologist's assistant: Basic rule and definitions. 42 CFR 410.7569-76. Retrieved from https://www.law.cornell.edu/cfr/text/42/410.69. (Accessed 7 September 2020.)

US Code of Federal Regulations. (2013). 42 CFR § 410.77 – Certified nurse-midwives' services: Qualifications and conditions. Retrieved from https://www.law.cornell.edu/cfr/text/42/410.77. (Accessed 7 September 2020.)

US Department of Veterans Affairs. (2017). Advanced practice registered nurse full practice authority. VHA Directive 1350. Retrieved from https://www.va.gov/vhapublications/publications.cfm?pub=1. (Accessed 7 September 2020.)

US Department of Veterans Affairs. (2018). Establishing medication prescribing authority for advanced practice nurses. VHA Directive 1075. Retrieved from https://www.va.gov/vhapublications/publications.cfm?pub=1. (Accessed 7 September 2020.)

Utah Controlled Substances Act Rules. (2019). Restrictions upon the prescription, dispensing and administration of controlled substances. R156-37-603. Retrieved from https://rules.utah.gov/publicat/code/r156/r156-37.htm#T15. (Accessed 7 September 2020.)

Washington Administrative Code 246-840-400. (2016) ARNP prescriptive authority. Retrieved from https://apps.leg.wa.gov/wac/default.aspx?cite=246-840-400. (Accessed 7 September 2020.)

Xue, Y., Ye, Z., Brewer, C., & Spetz, J. (2016). Impact of state nurse practitioner scope-of-practice regulation on health care delivery: Systematic review. *Nursing Outlook, 64*(1), 71–85.

Global Prescribing

5

Louise Kaplan

This chapter describes how and where registered nurse (RN) and advanced practice registered nurse (APRN) prescribing occurs. Many more countries permit RNs than APRNs to prescribe. There are different circumstances, such as task sharing or special training, and situations, such as high prevalence of human immunodeficiency virus (HIV) infections, under which RNs prescribe. APRN prescribing is more typically linked to initial education and regulation than is RN prescribing. As RN and APRN prescribing may be parallel processes, both are important to understand.

Advanced practice registered nurse (APRN) roles in the United States encompass nurse practitioners (NPs), certified nurse midwives (CNMs), clinical nurse specialists (CNSs), and certified registered nurse anesthetists (CRNAs). Several dozen countries have adopted one or more of the APRN roles, with the NP role the most common. In many countries, CNMs, CRNAs, and CNSs are not considered APRNs. Prescribing medication is a central element of APRN practice in the United States and is regulated by State Boards of Nursing. Globally, the regulation of APRN prescribing has slowly increased along with the expansion of APRNs. However, many countries still do not have a formal regulation process for APRN prescribers, which might prompt a discussion of the critical role that medications play in quality care.

As APRN prescribing has slowly increased, the ability of RNs to prescribe medication across the globe has also expanded, although the circumstances vary widely. While RNs in the United States are not allowed to prescribe, often they are able to implement a protocol to provide medication for a patient. Because the ability of RNs and APRNs to prescribe medication can be a parallel process, both are useful to understand as approaches to improving access to healthcare. An analysis of countries that have adopted APRN roles, APRN prescribing, and RN prescribing will inform a vision for the development and refinement of APRN scope of practice that includes the ability to prescribe medications. This chapter provides an overview of global RN and APRN prescribing and how these roles may co-exist.

The Advanced Practice Registered Nurse as a Prescriber, Second Edition. Edited by Louise Kaplan and Marie Annette Brown.
© 2021 John Wiley & Sons Ltd. Published 2021 by John Wiley & Sons Ltd.

DEFINING THE ADVANCED PRACTICE NURSE GLOBALLY

Scholarly articles typically refer to the definition of an advanced practice nurse (APN) that was developed by the International Council of Nurses (Andregard & Jangland, 2015; Delamaire & Lafortune 2010; Pan American Health Organization/ World Health Organization & McMaster University, 2017; Schober, 2016).

> A Nurse Practitioner/Advanced Practice Nurse is a registered nurse who has acquired the expert knowledge base, complex decision-making skills and clinical competencies for expanded practice, the characteristics of which are shaped by the context and/or country in which s/he is credentialed to practice. A master's level degree is recommended for entry level (International Council of Nurses [ICN], 2017).

Implementation of the definition of an APN varies widely among countries. The presence or absence of a regulatory framework has a major influence on nurses because it includes educational requirements, and definition and scope of practice for the APRN role (Gardner et al., 2016; Stasa et al., 2014). A total of 78 countries had the APN role in a 2020 global survey (World Health Organization, 2020c). The APRN role in the United States is distinct from other countries in how it clearly includes all four roles of CRNAs, CNMs, NPs, and CNSs. Considerable variability exists worldwide in which APRN roles are included in the definition of advanced practice.

Midwifery

In the United States, nurse midwifery began in 1925 when public health RNs educated in England began to provide perinatal care. Today, a graduate degree is required for entry into the nurse midwifery profession. However, in the United States and across the globe there is more than one pathway to midwifery. Several US states also recognize certified midwives and certified professional midwives who are not nurses (American College of Nurse-Midwives, 2020). In a survey of 58 countries, three pathways to midwifery were identified:

- Direct entry (no nursing education required)
- Midwifery as part of nursing education
- Post-nursing advanced education
  (Lal, 2014)

As an example, the Democratic Republic of Congo offers a three-year direct entry program for non-nurses or a one-year in-service program for nurses who have already completed a three-year nursing diploma program (Bogren et al., 2020).

Nurses as anesthesia providers

In the United States, the nurse anesthesia role was instituted in the late 1800s. CRNAs provide anesthesia care in every state and are the sole providers of anesthesia care in over 80% of rural counties (Martsolf et al., 2019). They play a similar and important role worldwide. In 1996, an international survey identified that nurses administered much or almost all anesthesia in at least 107 countries (McAuliffe & Henry, 1996). It is likely that the numbers and contributions of CRNAs have grown significantly since then.

Few countries recognize the CRNA as an APRN, primarily as education typically requires a certificate, although graduate education is being introduced. Educational requirements for CRNAs vary from a certificate program in the Democratic Republic of Congo, baccalaureate degree in Tunisia, master's degree in France, to a doctoral degree in the United States. The International Federation of Nurse Anesthetists (IFNA) has created a model core curriculum for both a certificate and master's program (IFNA, 2020).

Clinical nurse specialists
The first CNS role in the United States recognized psychiatric nursing as a specialty, with the first educational master's degree program established in 1954 (Lusk et al., 2019). In the 1970s the CNS role proliferated and developed in both depth and breadth, primarily in the hospital setting. CNSs practiced in multiple specialties such as oncology, women's health, critical care, and wound management (National Association of Clinical Nurse Specialists, 2020). The CNS role is now recognized in other countries such as Finland (ICN, 2018a), Canada, China, Hong Kong, Japan, New Zealand, the Republic of Korea, Taiwan, and the United Kingdom (Bryant-Lukosius & Wong, 2019). A graduate degree is required in Canada (Canadian Nurses Association, 2016), while in Hong Kong a nurse is appointed as a CNS as part of a clinical career pathway (Wong & Wong, 2020).

Nurse practitioners
The NP role was formally established in 1965 at the University of Colorado by Dr. Loretta Ford and Dr. Henry Silver. This pediatric NP certificate program prepared nurses to provide well-child and primary care for children. In subsequent decades, the NP role has evolved to encompass multiple specialties such as family practice, women's health, psychiatric mental-health, adult-gerontology primary care, adult-gerontology acute care, pediatric primary care, and pediatric acute care (Lusk et al., 2019). The NP role has disseminated worldwide.

COUNTRIES WITH ADVANCED PRACTICE ROLES
The definition of advanced practice and regulations for education and certification vary widely among the 78 countries with the APN role (WHO, 2020). This variability renders it difficult to determine the number of countries with an APN role congruent with the ICN definition. Nonetheless, the APN role has steadily expanded and is now widely adopted. Over a decade ago, Pulcini et al. (2010) identified 32 countries with 13 different titles; a subsequent survey identified only 26 countries with the APN role (Heale & Buckley, 2015).

Publications that describe the development of the APN role in a specific country help us better understand how the expansion process occurs and can inform the global nursing community about effective planning and implementation practices. For example, articles describe the development of APNs in Israel (Aaron & Andrews, 2016), Saudi Arabia (Hibbert et al., 2017), the United Arab Emirates (Behrens, 2018), and Norway (Ovrebo, 2018). Additional countries with emerging APN roles include Germany, Iceland, Sweden, Estonia,

Hungary (ICN, 2018b), Latvia, Lithuania, Luxembourg, Malta, Portugal, and Slovenia (Maier et al., 2017). The process of introduction and expansion of the APN role also varies. Hungary used a broad focus when it introduced six APRN roles including NPs and nurse anesthetists in 2017 through master's education. Eswatini (formerly known as Swaziland) instead introduced only the family nurse practitioner role (FNP) as a master's degree program (Anathan et al., 2020).

TASK SHARING

Task sharing is the process used to delegate responsibilities that require skill and knowledge from one group of health workers to another with different qualifications. This term, which is preferred over task-shifting, allows low-resourced countries with critical shortages of healthcare providers to expand and contract specific roles as needs change (Institute of Medicine, 2011). Typically, this realignment involves delegation of responsibilities from physicians to nurses or from licensed health professionals to community health workers, and may involve prescribing medication. Task sharing is both formal and informal, with and without authorization through nursing regulation (Christmals & Armstrong, 2019; Maier & Aiken, 2016). Task sharing is often part of a health system that may lack accountability and/or has limited ability to strengthen healthcare workers' competence to safely deliver care.

Task sharing is a strategy to deliver essential health services (WHO, 2008). Low-resourced countries typically have small health workforces and a high burden of disease. The African Region, for example, carries 22% of the global burden of disease, with 3% of the global health workforce and 1% of the world's financial resources (WHO, 2020b). These countries often carry a high burden of HIV infection so it is essential to increase access through antiretroviral therapies (ART). Consequently, nurses generally assume responsibility for people with illnesses such as HIV, tuberculosis (TB), malaria, non-communicable diseases, and childhood illnesses. This can save costs without compromising quality.

Task sharing is supported by strong evidence, the best of which relates to TB and HIV infection (Seidman & Atun, 2017). A study in South Africa compared outcomes for patients infected with HIV cared for by physicians and nurses. Time to initiation of ART and time to death did not differ between the groups, while viral load suppression was equivalent. Limitations of the study may have influenced why time to initiation of ART did not improve; however, the study supported the benefit of task sharing to nurses to improve access to care for people with HIV (Fairall et al., 2012).

The Global Alliance for Chronic Diseases (GACD) funded eight studies conducted to evaluate the effect of task sharing for the management of hypertension. In Argentina, Canada, Ghana, Kenya, South Africa, and Tanzania, the task sharing involved physicians and nurses. Based on research evidence, GACD affirmed the potential of task sharing to reduce premature morbidity and mortality related to cardiovascular disease (Joshi et al., 2018).

A qualitative study with 197 focus group participants in eight sub-Saharan African countries was conducted to establish role expectations of nurses and midwives. There was major disagreement whether nurses should diagnose and prescribe treatment including the prescription of medications. While viewed as life-saving in certain circumstances, such as when nurses work in remote areas, some stakeholders viewed this as nurses overstepping their boundaries (Seboni et al., 2013). Opposition was primarily from healthcare managers from Francophile countries.

Task sharing also occurs in well-resourced countries. Maier and Aiken (2016) examined the practice of task sharing from physicians to nurses, including APNs, in 39 well-resourced countries, of which 35 were European and the others were the United States, Canada, New Zealand and Australia, and the United Kingdom. Three clusters of countries emerged and were categorized as extensive, limited, or no task sharing. In the 11 countries with extensive task sharing, APNs assumed the responsibilities. In the 16 countries with limited task sharing, nurses, rather than APNs, assumed the tasks. No task sharing occurred in 12 countries.

Despite the best intentions, significant issues can arise when task sharing occurs. It can be resisted as an additional responsibility to an already overburdened healthcare worker who is not additionally remunerated (Joshi et al., 2018). Unfortunately, the inability of nurses to prescribe may limit the impact of task sharing (Joshi et al., 2018; Maier & Aiken, 2016).

NURSE PRESCRIBING

The ability to prescribe medications is one of the most essential elements of healthcare today. Prescribers, however, are generally in short supply outside of well-resourced countries. Task sharing from physicians to nurses that involves prescribing differs from the prescriptive authority given by regulatory bodies to nurses not prepared as APNs. In a survey of 320 regulatory jurisdictions across the world, 117 have at least one nursing role, including APNs and other nurses, with unrestricted prescriptive authority (National Council of State Boards of Nursing [NCSBN], 2020a). Table 5.1 provides an overview of different approaches to nurse prescribing.

Nurses may be independent prescribers or dependent and work under laws that require physician delegation or supervision (Maier, 2019). Within a country, some or all nurses may be authorized to prescribe, while the type of medications they can prescribe may range from a limited number to all drugs. Evidence supports nurse prescribing as an important contribution to global health, especially in regard to access to care. A systematic review concluded that nurse and physician prescribing were comparable in terms of the number of patients, number of medicines per patient visit, types and doses of medicines, and clinical outcomes with patients equally or more satisfied with the nurses' care (Gielen et al., 2014).

Prescribing by nurses is allowed in many countries with both dependent and independent models (Kooienga & Wilkinson, 2017). Australia permits nurse/midwife initiated medicines, which are non-prescription (over-the-counter), standing orders, and protocols (Australian Nursing & Midwifery Federation, 2018). In Europe alone, 13 countries legalized nurse prescribing. The type of medications, however, ranged from a limited set to nearly all medications within the nurse's area of practice. Nurses in Ireland, the United Kingdom, and

Table 5.1 Nurse prescribing within the nurse's specialty

Country	Title	Type of prescribing Initial/continuous*	Range/types of medications
Canada (Province of Alberta and approved in Ontario)	Registered nurse	Initial	Alberta: Prescribed medications that are not controlled substances Ontario: Proposal submitted to include vaccines, contraceptives, travel health, smoking cessation medication, over-the-counter medication, and epinephrine for anaphylaxis
Denmark	Registered nurse	Continuous	Vaccines, contraceptives, acute and chronic conditions, and pain medication
Eswatini	Registered nurse	Initial	Vitamins and minerals, vaccines, topical creams and ointments, most oral antibiotics and contraceptives, some pain medications and IV solutions
Finland	Nurse prescriber	Initial and continuous	Initial: Vaccines, hormonal contraception, certain acute illnesses, local anesthetics Continuous: Chronic conditions
Ireland	Nurse prescriber	Initial	Vaccines, contraceptives, acute and chronic conditions, and pain medication
Poland	RN (master's degree) RN (bachelor's degree)	Master's educated: Initial Baccalaureate educated: Continuous	Ministry of Health has designated over 30 medications including contraceptives, asthma, throat, ear, sinus, UTI, analgesics and locally acting anesthetics, antiemetics, antiparasitics, IV fluids
Netherlands	Nurse specialist	Initial	Medications for diabetes, and pulmonary and oncology chronic conditions and pain medication for oncology
	Specialist nurses in diabetes, lung, oncology	Continuous	Protocol use required after initial diagnosis by a physician
South Africa	Professional nurse	Initial	Full range of medications for all conditions that are in the STG-EML
Timor-Leste	Registered nurse	Initial	Essential Medicines List for use in community health centers including some antibiotics, antimalarials, and contraceptives; topical creams and ointments, vaccines, and oral rehydration therapy
United Kingdom	Registered nurse	Initial if independent	Independent prescriber: All medications including some controlled substances. Supplementary prescriber:
	Independent and supplementary	Continuous if supplementary	Limited based on a clinical management plan for the patient

*Initial prescribing is for a new medication/product and continued prescriptions whereas continuous prescribing is follow-up after a physician provides the initial prescription. STG-EML, Standard Treatment Guidelines and Essential Medicines List; UTI, urinary tract infection.

some in the Netherlands have full prescribing rights within their specialty (Maier, 2019).

Standard treatment guidelines (STGs) and essential medication lists (EMLs) are a critical facilitator for nurse-led care because they allow and guide nurses to prescribe medications. This option is utilized in countries such as Eswatini, South Africa, and Timor-Leste (Republica Democratica de Timor-Leste Ministerio Da Saude, 2010; Republic of South Africa Department: Health, 2018; Sooruth et al., 2015; Swaziland Ministry of Health, 2012). STGs provide evidence-based recommendations for preventive care and treatment for common problems in a country to improve quality of care. STGs incorporate the appropriate use of drugs contained in the EML. Since 1977, WHO has regularly updated and published a model EML formulary to provide guidance to countries and healthcare professionals for the purchase, supply, and use of medications in the public sector (WHO, 2020a). In Eswatini, the EML allows both RNs and doctors to prescribe level A drugs such as vitamins and minerals, vaccines, topical creams and ointments, most oral antibiotics and contraceptives, and many IV solutions. RNs in Eswatini may also participate in a nurse-led program to initiate antiretroviral treatment for people with HIV infection after a five-day didactic course and a five-day clinical practicum (Mavhandu-Mudzusi et al., 2017).

Examples of requirements and the scope of nurse prescribing follow. In the subsequent section, examples of the requirements and scope of APRN prescribing are included to allow for comparison, showing the similarities and differences between nurse and APRN prescribing.

United Kingdom

The nurse prescriber role in the United Kingdom was formally approved in 2002 as either an independent or supplementary role; full implementation, however, did not occur until 2006 (Dowden, 2016; Graham-Clarke et al., 2019). Subsequent legislative changes meant that nurse prescribers in the UK have the greatest prescribing authority in the world. They can prescribe virtually all drugs, including controlled drugs (Dowden, 2016).

There are certain requirements for a nurse to obtain prescriptive authority. These include completing a training program in their specified clinical field (e.g. mental health), having at least three years of practice experience, and being deemed competent to prescribe by their employer (Dowden, 2016). Two categories of nurse prescribers exist, independent and supplementary. The independent nurse prescriber is accountable for care of the patient including assessment, diagnosis, management, and prescribing. The supplementary nurse prescriber manages conditions and prescribes medications listed in an agreed clinical management plan which is initiated by a physician (Graham-Clarke et al., 2019).

Poland

In January 2016, Poland authorized nurses to prescribe. They may also refer patients for diagnostic tests and complete a physical examination prior to prescribing (WHO, 2020d). A baccalaureate-educated nurse who completes an appropriate specialist course may become a supplementary prescriber and continue a patient's treatment as initiated by a physician. A nurse with a master's degree or specialty and an appropriate specialist course may prescribe medications as an independent nurse prescriber and initiate medications (Zarzeka et al., 2017). The Ministry of Health selected over 30 medications and some medical devices, such as blood glucose monitoring equipment, which may be nurse prescribed.

Ireland

Ireland in 2007 authorized nurses to independently prescribe medications within the scope of their clinical practice upon completion of a six-month post-graduate course (Wilson et al., 2018). There are basic requirements prior to the actual educational prescribing program. These include a minimum of three years of relevant clinical experience, having employer support, and meeting national competencies equivalent to baccalaureate education to be eligible to complete an educational prescribing program. The program has both classroom and practicum components. Commonly prescribed medications include paracetamol and ibuprofen, vaccines, contraceptives, antibiotics, and medication for acute and chronic illnesses (Maier, 2019; Wilson et al., 2018).

Canada

In Canada, only the province of Alberta has RN prescribing, implemented in May 2019. Nurses must have at least 3,000 hours of practice as an RN, with at least 750 of them in the practice setting/location where the RN will prescribe, complete an RN prescribing course, and have employer support. RNs who qualify may prescribe Schedule I drugs, which in Canada refers to all typically prescribed medications except controlled drugs (College and Association of Registered Nurses of Alberta, 2019). Nurse prescribing is intended for use with a patient whose condition is stable.

Ontario legislation passed in 2017 allowed the College of Nurses of Ontario to develop regulations for RNs to prescribe; however, implementation has not occurred at the time of this writing. The College intends to allow RNs to prescribe immunizations, contraceptives, medications for travel health and smoking cessation, over-the-counter medications, and epinephrine for anaphylaxis (College of Nurses of Ontario, 2019a).

OUTCOMES OF NURSE PRESCRIBING

A study of nurses working in primary healthcare clinics in the South African province of KwaZulu-Natal revealed they prescribed according to the STGs and EML with no evidence of polypharmacy. The process of prescription writing itself was suboptimal and related to insufficient training (Sooruth et al., 2015). In Namibia, a review of 1,090 prescriptions indicated medical officers prepared 37.5%, registered nurses/midwives prepared 32%, and enrolled nurses/midwives 25.8%. Evaluation of the prescriptions for adherence to the STGs revealed medical officers complied 27.7%, enrolled nurses/midwives, 27%, and registered nurses/midwives 22.6% of the time (Akpabio et al., 2015).

Botswana addressed its HIV epidemic in the 1990s and trained health professionals, including nurses, to prescribe ART. The Ministry of Health and the Harvard AIDS Institute Partnership developed a training program referred to as KITSO (knowledge innovation and training shall overcome AIDS). Within four years, 90% of people who needed ART were on treatment and received follow-up care (WHO, 2015). A study that compared the performance of physician and nurse prescribers caring for HIV-infected children reviewed documentation of eight clinically relevant aspects of care. Nurse prescribers and physicians correctly documented 96.0% and 94.9% of the time respectively. The data suggested that nurses provided more social history and demonstrated higher effectiveness compared to physicians in their approach to the ART protocols (Monyatsi et al., 2012).

APRN PRESCRIBING

Development of the APRN role across the globe has been accompanied by a patchwork of regulations. Six countries allow nurse prescribing only at the advanced practice level and require a minimum of a master's degree education (Ladd & Schober, 2018). In many countries, prescribing is not a component of advanced practice nursing; not all countries with the APRN role even regulate advanced practice. For example, Jamaica regulates the NP and nurse anesthetist role, although independent prescribing is not included in the scope of practice and requires a physician's co-signature (ICN, 2017). Most APRN prescribing occurs in European and North American countries; however, other countries such as Australia and New Zealand also authorize APRN prescribing (Ladd & Schober, 2018). Examples of APRN prescribing follow.

Australia

Advanced practice nursing in Australia recognizes and regulates only the NP role. NPs began practice in Australia in 2000, with prescribing authority authorized a year later. To date, there were 1,929 NPs in the country (Nursing and Midwifery Board of Australia [NMBA], 2020). Medications are classified into ten schedules. Schedules 2, 3, 4, and 8 include medicinal substances intended for human therapeutic use (Australian Government Department of Health Therapeutic Goods Administration, 2019). Each state and territory determines whether there is blanket NP prescribing authority or if restrictions exist, such as prescribing based on the use of a formulary (NMBA, 2016). Two of the states with large numbers of NPs are Victoria and New South Wales.

NPs in Victoria may obtain, possess, use, supply, or prescribe Schedule 2, 3, 4, or 8 medications approved by the Minister of Health. The list of approved drugs is specific to each category of NP. These categories include acute and supportive care, care of the older person or aged care, critical care, maternity care, mental health care, pediatric care, perioperative care, and primary care. The NP in primary care has a broad list of approved medications that range from anticoagulants, antihypertensives, antibiotics, and insulin to narcotic analgesics, antiretrovirals, and hypnotics (Victoria State Government, 2020).

Beginning March 2020, all NPs in New South Wales, whether employed in the private or public sector, may possess, use, supply, and/or prescribe any

Schedule 2, 3, 4, or 8 medication within the NP's scope of practice (NSW Government, 2020). There are certain medications that may only be prescribed by a clinician who has a separate endorsement. For example, prescribing alprazolam or flunitrazepam to a person for more than two months requires special authorization (NSW Government, 2018).

A comprehensive review of Australian NP prescribing revealed that some consumers were unaware of NP prescriptive authority and that some health professionals still had reservations about NP prescribing (Fong et al., 2017). Analgesics and anti-infective medications were the most frequently prescribed. NPs were most confident when they provided education about medication, although as years of experience increased, their confidence with medication management also increased.

Canada

Every province and territory in Canada recognizes and regulates NPs. Their main role is the provision of direct patient care, including primary care in both physician and NP-led practices and community clinics and health centers, long-term care, and some areas of hospitals (Canadian Nurses Association, 2020a). CNSs in Canada work at the client, practice setting, and systems levels. Their main focus is to improve clinical excellence and support implementation of evidence-based practice rather than provide direct patient care (Canadian Nurses Association, 2020b).

NPs have a legally authorized scope of practice to diagnose, order, and interpret diagnostic tests, prescribe medications and other treatments, and perform procedures within their legislated scope (Canadian Nurses Association, 2019). NPs are educated and registered for family, adult, pediatric, neonatal, cardiology, nephrology, and primary care practice. All jurisdictions authorize prescriptive authority which includes controlled drugs and substances, with limits in the Yukon and Quebec. Federal restrictions for controlled drugs and substances prescribing were removed in 2012 which afforded the provinces the opportunity to complete NP prescribing. Ontario was an early regulator of the NP role, while British Columbia was one of the last provinces to implement NP legislation. Often states with a higher density of physicians, like British Columbia, offer the greatest resistance to a full scope of practice for NPs.

In Ontario, NPs may prescribe, dispense, compound, sell, or administer substances by injection and inhalation, although controlled drugs may not be sold or compounded. Certain conditions are specified about these activities. An approved education course must be successfully completed to prescribe controlled substances; however, opium, coca leaves and anabolic steroids other than testosterone are explicitly excluded. NPs must follow guidelines and restrictions in order to prescribe, dispense, compound, and sell controlled drugs. For example, an NP may only compound a controlled drug if the client does not have reasonable or timely access to a pharmacy, would not otherwise receive the medication, or does not have the financial resources to obtain the medication if it is not compounded by the NP (College of Nurses of Ontario, 2019b).

NPs in British Columbia may prescribe medications, including controlled drugs, with certain restrictions. They may also compound, administer, and dispense any medication they can prescribe. Restrictions include, but are not limited to, specific education requirements that must be met to prescribe for specific classifications or situations. These include antiretroviral drugs for the prevention or treatment of HIV infection; cancer treatment drugs; controlled drugs; and methadone for analgesia. Other restrictions limit the use of certain amphetamines only for designated conditions and do not allow general anesthetics to induce general anesthesia (British Columbia College of Nursing Professionals, 2020).

New Zealand
New Zealand first recognized the NP role in 2001 and has a regulated scope of practice including prescriptive authority. The CNS role is not regulated, qualifications vary at the discretion of the employer, and there is confusion about the role (Carryer et al., 2018). In a national survey, more respondents identified as a CNS than an NP, with many similarities in domains of care. Many CNSs who are eligible for NP licensure do not apply, as NP positions are lacking despite a defined NP scope of practice. NPs compete for positions with other nursing roles designated in the country's healthcare system's collective bargaining agreement (Carryer et al., 2018). Midwives and anesthetists are not considered advanced practice nursing roles (New Zealand College of Midwives, n.d.; Perioperative Nurses College, 2014).

In 2017, the Nursing Council of New Zealand adopted new guidelines to allow NPs to self-regulate and practice in their areas of competence and experience, rather than a specific area of practice (Nursing Council of New Zealand, 2019). They are authorized to prescribe any medication relevant to their area of practice and issue standing orders for RNs to administer and/or supply medications to assure patients experience timely access to medication. The standing order excludes the generation of a prescription to be dispensed at a pharmacy (Ministry of Health, 2016). NPs can prescribe controlled drugs and classes A, B, and C. The classes reflect potential level of harm. Class A drugs are very high risk, class B drugs are high risk of harm, and class C drugs are moderate risk of harm (New Zealand Legislation, 2019). These include but are not limited to opioids, benzodiazepines, and stimulants. NPs may not prescribe controlled drugs for addiction treatment (Ministry of Health, 2013). One retrospective study evaluated NP prescribing patterns between 2013 and 2015, at a time when not all NPs were required to register to prescribe. The study found that 129 of 145 NPs prescribed at least one medication during the study period. There were 603 different medications prescribed across six specialties, with paracetamol and amoxicillin the top two prescribed medications (Poot et al., 2017).

United Kingdom
Advanced practice nursing in the UK is limited to the NP role, titled Advanced Nurse Practitioner (ANP). The first students graduated from a formal NP academic program in 1992, with initial guidance on the role provided in 1996

by the Royal College of Nursing (RCN, 2008). By 2006, APNs were able to prescribe. Standards developed for advanced level nursing practice in 2018 require a master's degree with advanced pharmacology and evidence-based prescribing to qualify as an independent prescriber (RCN, 2018).

In the UK, the APN practices in an autonomous role and cares for people with undifferentiated problems and long-term health conditions (Bayless-Pratt & Gregory, 2017). As independent prescribers, APNs have been able to prescribe any medication in the British National Formulary since 2006 (RCN, 2014). Since 2012 they may prescribe controlled drugs in Schedules 2–5 when clinically appropriate and within the scope of practice, with a few exclusions (RCN, 2019). Examples of medications that are allowed are Schedule 2 drugs such as opioids and stimulants. Schedule 3 drugs include buprenorphine, phenteramine, and temazepam, Schedule 4 drugs are primarily benzodiazepines, while Schedule 5 drugs include some preparations of certain controlled drugs in low strengths, such as codeine preparations (The National Archives, 2001).

United States
APRN prescribing is authorized in all 50 states for NPs and CNMs. CRNAs are unable to prescribe in 14 states, and CNSs are unable to prescribe in 16 states (NCSBN, 2020b). Even in states that authorize APRNs to prescribe, laws vary widely. States with full practice authority have no restrictions, although in some states prescribing is limited to the area of certification and licensure. States with reduced or restricted practice may require a protocol, use of a formulary, practice agreement, or delegation of prescribing authority by a physician. Chapter 4 provides an in-depth overview of APRN prescribing in the United States.

CONCLUSION
APRN prescribing that includes all four APRN roles (NPs, CNSs, CRNAs, and CNMs) is confined to the United States. APRN prescribing globally is usually limited to NPs and sometimes includes CNMs. Nurse prescribing is more widespread across the globe than APRN prescribing. Likely factors include slow evolution of APRN education and practice; limited formal regulation which would define the scope of practice for APRNs; and a need for greater access to care that is provided by the substantial nursing workforce and task sharing. It is also likely that nurse prescribers may be resistant to the expansion of APRN prescribing in countries where nurses hold a key role as prescribers. As APRN roles evolve, a useful strategy to strengthen the profession will be to advocate for regulation inclusive of prescriptive authority and collaboration among all nurses to enhance access to care.

REFERENCES
Aaron, E.M., & Andrews, C.S. (2016). Integration of advanced practice providers into the Israeli healthcare system. *Israel Journal of Health Policy Research, 5*(7), 1–18.

Akpabio, E., Sagwa, E., Mazibuko, G., et al. (2015). Assessment of compliance of outpatient prescribing with the Namibia Standard Treatment Guidelines

in public sector health facilities. Retrieved from http://siapsprogram.org/
publication/assessment-of-compliance-of-outpatient-prescribing-with-the-
namibia-standard-treatment-guidelines-in-public-sector-health-facilities/f.
(Accessed 7 September 2020.)

American College of Nurse-Midwives. (2020). Comparison of certified nurse-
midwives, certified midwives, certified professional midwives clarifying the
distinctions among professional midwifery credentials in the U.S. Retrieved from
http://www.midwife.org/acnm/files/cclibraryfiles/filename/000000007045/
final-comparisonchart-oct2017.pdf. (Accessed 7 September 2020.)

Anathan, J., Dlamini, C.P., & Kaplan, L. (2020). Developing advanced practice
nursing education, practice and policy in Eswatini. In S. Hassmiller & J.
Pulcini (Eds), *Advanced practice nursing leadership: A global perspective*. New
York: Springer Nature.

Andregard, A.-C., & Jangland, E. (2015). The tortuous journey of introducing
the nurse practitioner as a new member of the healthcare team: A meta-syn-
thesis. *Scandinavian Journal of Caring Sciences, 29*, 3–14.

Australian Government Department of Health Therapeutic Goods
Administration. (2019). Scheduling handbook: guidance for amending the
Poisons Standard. Retrieved from https://www.tga.gov.au/publication/
scheduling-handbook-guidance-amending-poisons-standard. (Accessed 7
September 2020.)

Australian Nursing & Midwifery Federation. (2018). Registered nurse and
midwife prescribing. ANMF position statement. Retrieved from http://
www.anmf.org.au/documents/policies/p_registered_nurse_and_midwife_
prescribing.pdf. (Accessed 7 September 2020.)

Bayless-Pratt, L., & Gregory, S. (2017). The general practice nursing workforce
development plan. Health Education England. Retrieved from https://
www.hee.nhs.uk/sites/default/files/documents/The%20general%20
practice%20nursing%20workforce%20development%20plan.pdf. (Accessed
7 September 2020.)

Behrens, S.A. (2018). Constructing an advanced practice registered nurse practice
model in the UAE: Using innovation to address cultural implications and challenges in an international enterprise. *Nursing Administration Quarterly, 42*(1), 83–90.

Bogren, M., Ndela, B., Toko, C., & Berg, M. (2020). Midwifery education, regulation and association in the Democratic Republic of Congo (DRC) – current
state and challenges. *Global Health Action, 13*(1), 1–9.

British Columbia College of Nursing Professionals. (2020). NP Scope of practice.
Retrieved from https://www.bccnp.ca/standards/rn_np/npscopepractice/
pages/default.aspx. (Accessed 7 September 2020.)

Bryant-Lukosius, D., & Wong, F.K.Y. (2019). International development of
advanced practice nursing. In M.F. Tracy, & E.T. O'Grady (Eds), *Hamric and
Hanson's advanced practice nursing: An integrative review* (pp. 129–141).
Amsterdam: Elsevier.

Canadian Nurses Association. (2016). Clinical nurse specialist: Position statement.
Retrieved from https://www.cna-aiic.ca/-/media/cna/page-content/pdf-en/
clinical-nurse-specialist-position-statement_2016.pdf?la=en&hash=c89816295fe2
f53808e0dedc0595fe376552eae1. (Accessed 7 September 2020.)

Canadian Nurses Association. (2019). Advanced practice nursing: A Pan-Canadian framework. Retrieved from https://cna-aiic.ca/-/media/cna/page-content/pdf-en/advanced-practice-nursing-framework-en.pdf?la=en&hash=76a98adee62e655e158026deb45326c8c9528b1b. (Accessed 7 September 2020.)

Canadian Nurses Association. (2020a). Nurse practitioners. Retrieved from https://cna-aiic.ca/en/nursing-practice/the-practice-of-nursing/advanced-nursing-practice/nurse-practitioners. (Accessed 7 September 2020.)

Canadian Nurses Association. (2020b). Clinical nurse specialists. Retrieved from https://cna-aiic.ca/en/nursing-practice/the-practice-of-nursing/advanced-nursing-practice/clinical-nurse-specialists. (Accessed 7 September 2020.)

Carryer, J., Wilkinson, J., Towers, A., & Gardner, G. (2018). Delineating advanced practice nursing in New Zealand: A national survey. *International Nursing Review, 65*(1), 24–32.

Christmals, C.D., & Armstrong, S.J. (2019). The essence, opportunities and threats to advanced practice nursing in Sub-Saharan Africa: A scoping review. *Heliyon, 5*(10), 1–21.

College and Association of Registered Nurses of Alberta. (2019). Registered nurses prescribing schedule 1 drugs and ordering diagnostic tests. Retrieved from https://nurses.ab.ca/docs/default-source/document-library/standards/registered-nurse-prescribing-schedule-1-drugs-and-ordering-diagnostic-tests-requirements-and-standards.pdf?sfvrsn=67eba52b_14. (Accessed 7 September 2020.)

College of Nurses of Ontario. (2019a). FAQs: RN prescribing. Retrieved from https://www.cno.org/en/trending-topics/journey-to-rn-prescribing/qas-rn-prescribing/. (Accessed 7 September 2020.)

College of Nurses of Ontario. (2019b). Practice standard: Nurse practitioner. Retrieved from https://www.cno.org/globalassets/docs/prac/41038_strdrnec.pdf. (Accessed 7 September 2020.)

Delamaire, M., & Lafortune, G. (2010). *Nurses in advanced roles: A description and evaluation of experiences in 12 developed countries.* OECD Health Working Papers, No. 54. Paris: OECD Publishing.

Dowden, A. (2016). The expanding role of nurse prescribers. Retrieved from https://www.prescriber.co.uk/article/expanding-role-nurse-prescribers/. (Accessed 7 September 2020.)

Fairall, L., Bachmann, M.O., Lombard, C., et al. (2012). Task shifting of antiretroviral treatment from doctors to primary care nurses in South Africa (STRETCH): a pragmatic, parallel, cluster-randomised trial. *Lancet, 380,* 889–980.

Fong, J., Buckley, T., Cashin, A., & Pont, L. (2017). Nurse practitioner prescribing in Australia: A comprehensive literature review. *Australia Critical Care, 30,* 252–259.

Gardner, G., Duffield, C., Doubrovsky, A., & Adams, A. (2016). Identifying advanced practice: A national survey of a nursing workforce. *International Journal of Nursing Studies, 55,* 60–70.

Gielen, S.C., Dekker, J., Francke, A.L., et al. (2014). The effects of nurse prescribing: A systematic review. *International Journal of Nursing Studies, 51,* 1048–1061.

Graham-Clarke, E., Rushton, A., Noblet, T., & Marriott, J. (2019). Non-medical prescribing in the United Kingdom National Health Service: A systematic policy review. *PLoS ONE, 14*(7), e0214630.

Heale, R., & Buckley, C.R. (2015). An international perspective of advanced practice nursing regulation. *International Nursing Review, 62*(3), 421–429.

Hibbert, D., Aboshaiqah, A.E., Sienko, K.A., et al. (2017). Advancing nursing practice: The emergence of the role of advanced practice nurse in Saudi Arabia. *Annals of Saudi Medicine, 37*(1), 72–78.

Higuchi, M., Okumura, J., Aoyama, A., et al. (2015). Use of medications and adherence to standard treatment guidelines in rural community health centers, Timor-Leste. *Asia-Pacific Journal of Public Health, 27*(2), NP2498–NP2511.

Institute of Medicine. (2011). *Preparing for the future of HIV? AIDS in Africa: A shared responsibility.* Washington, DC: The National Academies Press.

International Council of Nurses. (2017). Country specific practice profiles: Jamaica. Retrieved from https://international.aanp.org/content/docs/jamaica.pdf. (Accessed 7 September 2020.)

International Council of Nurses. (2018a). Country specific practice profiles: Finland. Retrieved from https://international.aanp.org/content/docs/finland.pdf. (Accessed 7 September 2020.)

International Council of Nurses. (2018b). Country specific practice profiles: Interest in advanced practice nursing in Hungary. Retrieved from https://international.aanp.org/content/docs/hungary.pdf. (Accessed 7 September 2020.)

Joshi, R., Thrift, A.G., Smith, C., et al. (2018). Task-shifting for cardiovascular risk factor management: lessons from the Global Alliance for Chronic Disease. *BMJ Global Health, 3*(Suppl 3), e001092.

Kooienga, S., & Wilkinson, J. (2017). RN prescribing: An expanded role for nursing. *Nursing Forum, 52*(1), 3–11.

Ladd, E., & Shober, M. (2018). Nurse prescribing from the global vantage point: The intersection between role and policy. *Policy, Politics, & Nursing Practice, 191*(1–2), 40–49.

Lal, G. (2014). Comprehensive midwifery programme guidance. Retrieved from https://www.unfpa.org/sites/default/files/resource-pdf/midwifery%20programme%20guidance.pdf. (Accessed 7 September 2020.)

Lusk, B., Cockerham, A.Z., & Keeling, A.W. (2019). Highlights from the history of advanced practice nursing in the United States. In M.F. Tracy, & E.T. O'Grady (Eds), *Hamric and Hanson's advanced practice nursing: An integrative review* (pp. 1–24). Amsterdam: Elsevier.

Maier, C. (2019). Nurse prescribing of medicines in 13 European countries. *Human Resources for Health, 17*(95).

Maier, C.B., & Aiken, L.H. (2016). Task shifting from physicians to nurses in primary care in 39 countries: A cross-country comparative study. *European Journal of Public Health, 26*(6), 927–934.

Maier, C., Aiken, L., & Busse, R. (2017). *Nurses in advanced roles in primary care: Policy levers for implementation.* OECD Health Working Papers, No. 98. Paris: OECD Publishing.

Martsolf, G.R., Baird, M., Cohen, C.C., & Koirala, N. (2019). Relationship between state policy and anesthesia provider supply in rural communities. *Medical Care, 57*(5), 341–347.

Mavhandu-Mudzusi, A.H., Sandy, P.T., & Hettema, L. (2017). Registered nurses' perception regarding nurse-led antiretroviral therapy initiation in Hhohho region, Swaziland. *International Nursing Review, 64*, 552–560.

McAuliffe, M.S., & Henry, B. (1996). Countries where anesthesia is administered by nurses. *Journal of the American Association of Nurse Anesthetists, 64*(5), 469–479.

Midwives Australia. (n.d.) For students. Retrieved from http://www.midwivesaustralia.com.au/?page_id=72. (Accessed 7 September 2020.)

Ministry of Health. (2013). *Prescribing controlled drugs in addiction treatment: Section 24 Misuse of Drugs Act 1975*. Wellington: Ministry of Health.

Ministry of Health. (2016). *Standing order guidelines*, 2nd ed. Wellington: Ministry of Health.

Monyatsi, G., Mullam, P.C., Phelps, B.R., et al. (2012). HIV management by nurse prescribers compared with doctors at a paediatric center in Gaborone, Botswana. *South African Medical Journal, 100*(6).

National Association of Clinical Nurse Specialists. (2020). What is a CNS? Retrieved from https://nacns.org/about-us/what-is-a-cns/. (Accessed 7 September 2020.)

National Council of State Boards of Nursing. (2020a). A global profile of nursing regulation, education, and practice. *Journal of Nursing Regulation, 10*(Special Issue), 1–117.

National Council of State Boards of Nursing. (2020b). Member board profiles: 2019 advanced practice registered nurse survey. Retrieved from https://www.ncsbn.org/2019aprn.pdf. (Accessed 7 September 2020.)

New Zealand College of Midwives. (n.d.). How to become a midwife. Retrieved from https://www.midwife.org.nz/midwives/midwifery-in-new-zealand/how-to-become-a-midwife/.

New Zealand Legislation. (2019). Misuse of Drugs Act 1975: Classification of drugs. Retrieved from http://www.legislation.govt.nz/act/public/1975/0116/latest/DLM436190.html. (Accessed 7 September 2020.)

NSW Government. (2018). Upscaling of alprazolam from schedule 4 to schedule 8. Retrieved from https://www.health.nsw.gov.au/pharmaceutical/pages/alprazolam-upscheduling.aspx. (Accessed 7 September 2020.)

NSW Government. (2020). Nurse practitioners in NSW. Retrieved from https://www.health.nsw.gov.au/nursing/practice/pages/nurse-practitoner.aspx. (Accessed 7 September 2020.)

Nursing and Midwifery Board of Australia. (2016). Safety and quality guidelines for nurse practitioners. Retrieved from https://www.nursingmidwiferyboard.gov.au/codes-guidelines-statements/codes-guidelines/safety-and-quality-guidelines-for-nurse-practitioners.aspx. (Accessed 7 September 2020.)

Nursing and Midwifery Board of Australia. (2020). Registrant data. Retrieved from https://www.nursingmidwiferyboard.gov.au/search.aspx?q=registrant+data. (Accessed 7 September 2020.)

Nursing Council of New Zealand. (2019). Nurse practitioner scope of practice. Retrieved from https://www.nursingcouncil.org.nz/public/nursing/scopes_of_practice/nurse_practitioner/ncnz/nursing-section/nurse_practitioner.aspx. (Accessed 7 September 2020.)

Ovrebo, A. (2018). The challenges and advantages of advanced nurse practitioners in Norwegian community healthcare, as experienced by nurse managers. Retrieved from https://openarchive.usn.no/usn-xmlui/bitstream/handle/11250/2629247/locked_until_20200101master%c3%98vreb%c3%b82018.pdf?sequence=1. (Accessed 7 September 2020.)

Pan American Health Organization/World Health Organization, McMaster University. (2017). Report: Universal access to health and universal health coverage: advanced practice nursing summit. Retrieved from http://www.observatoriorh.org/?q=report-universal-access-health-and-universal-health-coverage-advanced-practice-nursing-summit. (Accessed 7 September 2020.)

Perioperative Nurses College. (2014). Frequently asked questions: Nurse assistant to the anaesthetist. Retrieved from https://www.nzno.org.nz/portals/0/files/documents/groups/perioperative%20nurses/faq%20nurses%20assistant%20to%20the%20anaesthetist%20may%202014.pdf. (Accessed 7 September 2020.)

Poot, B., Zonneveld, R., Nelson, K., & Weatherall, M. (2017). Prescribing by nurse practitioners: Insight from a New Zealand study. *Journal of the American Association of Nurse Practitioners*, 29, 581–590.

Pulcini, J., Jelic, M., Gul, R., & Loke, A.Y. (2010). An international survey on advanced practice nursing education, practice, and regulation. *Journal of Nursing Scholarship*, 42(1), 31–39.

Republic of South Africa Department: Health. (2018). Standard treatment guidelines and essential medicines list for South Africa: Primary healthcare level. Retrieved from https://www.idealhealthfacility.org.za/docs/guidelines/stg%20and%20eml%20phc%202018.pdf. (Accessed 7 September 2020.)

Republica Democratica de Timore-Leste Ministerio Da Saude. (2010). Essential medicines list for Timor-Leste 2010. Retrieved from http://www.moh.gov.tl/?q=node/165. (Accessed 7 September 2020.)

Royal College of Nursing. (2008). Advanced nurse practitioners – an RCN guide to the advanced nurse practitioner role, competencies and programme accreditation. Retrieved from http://aape.org.uk/wp-content/uploads/2015/02/rcn-anp-guidance-document-2008.pdf. (Accessed 7 September 2020.)

Royal College of Nursing. (2014). RCN factsheet on nurse prescribing in the UK. Retrieved from https://www.rcn.org.uk/about-us/policy-briefings/pol-1512. (Accessed 7 September 2020.)

Royal College of Nursing. (2018). RCN standards for advanced level nursing practice. Retrieved from https://www.rcn.org.uk/professional-development/publications/pub-007038. (Accessed 7 September 2020.)

Royal College of Nursing. (2019). Non-medical prescribers: Nurse independent prescribers and controlled drugs. Retrieved from https://www.rcn.org.uk/get-help/rcn-advice/non-medical-prescribers. (Accessed 7 September 2020.)

Schober, M. (2016). *Introduction to advanced practice nursing: An international focus.* Cham: Springer Nature Switzerland.

Seboni, N.M., Magowe, M.K.M., Uys, L.R., et al. (2013). Shaping the role of sub-Saharan African nurses and midwives: Stakeholder's perceptions of the nurses' and midwives' tasks and roles. *Health SA Gesondheid 18*(1), 1–11.

Seidman, G., & Atun, R. (2017). Does task shifting yield cost savings and improve efficiency for health systems? A systematic review of evidence from low-income and middle-income countries. *Human Resources for Health, 15*(29).

Sooruth, U.R., Sibiya, M.N., & Sokhela, D.G. (2015). The use of standard treatment guidelines and essential medicine list by professional nurses at primary healthcare clinics in uMgungundlovu District in South Africa. *International Journal of Africa Nursing Sciences, 3*, 50–55.

Stasa, H., Cashin, A., Buckley, T., & Donoghue, J. (2014). Advancing advanced practice – Clarifying the conceptual confusion. *Nursing Education Today, 34*(3), 356–361.

Swaziland Ministry of Health. (2012). Standard treatment guidelines and essential medicines list of common medical conditions in the Kingdom of Swaziland. Retrieved from https://apps.who.int/medicinedocs/documents/s22119en/s22119en.pdf. (Accessed 7 September 2020.)

Tanzania Ministry of Health, Community Development, Gender, Elderly and Children. (2017). *Standard treatment guidelines and national essential medicines list. Tanzania mainland.* Retrieved from http://www.tzdpg.or.tz/fileadmin/documents/dpg_internal/dpg_working_groups_clusters/cluster_2/health/key_sector_documents/tanzania_key_health_documents/standard_treatment_guidelines__correct_final_use_this-1.pdf. (Accessed 7 September 2020.)

The National Archives. (2001). The misuse of drugs regulations 2001. Retrieved from http://www.legislation.gov.uk/uksi/2001/3998/contents/made. (Accessed 7 September 2020.)

Victoria State Government. (2020). Approved by the Minister of Health. Retrieved from https://www2.health.vic.gov.au/public-health/drugs-and-poisons/drugs-poisons-legislation/approved-by-the-minister. (Accessed 7 September 2020.)

Wilson, D.M., Murphy, J., Nam, M.A., et al. (2018). Nurse and midwifery prescribing in Ireland: A scope-of-practice development for worldwide consideration. *Nursing and Health Sciences, 20*, 264–270.

Wong, F.K.Y., & Wong, A.K.C. (2020). Advanced practice nursing in Hong Kong and Mainland China. In S.B. Hassmiller & J. Pulcini (Eds), *Advanced practice nursing leadership: A global perspective.* New York: Springer Nature.

World Health Organization. (2008). *Task shifting: rational redistribution of tasks among healthcare teams: global recommendations and guidelines.* Geneva: WHO.

World Health Organization. (2015). Realizing nurses' full potential. *Bulletin of the World Health Organization, 93*(9), 596–597.

World Health Organization. (2020a). Strengthening access to essential medicines. Retrieved from https://www.who.int/activities/strengthening-access-to-essential-medicines. (Accessed 7 September 2020.)

World Health Organization. (2020b). Global health observatory (GHO) data: Density of medical doctors. Retrieved from https://www.who.int/gho/health_workforce/doctors_density/en/. (Accessed 7 September 2020.)

World Health Organization. (2020c). State of the world's nursing: Investing in education, jobs, and leadership. Retrieved from https://www.who.int/publications-detail/nursing-report-2020. (Accessed 7 September 2020.)

World Health Organization. (2020d). Improving access to medicines in primary care: Nurse prescribing in Poland. Retrieved from http://www.euro.who.int/__data/assets/pdf_file/0006/441915/case-study-nurse-prescribing.pdf?ua=1. (Accessed 7 September 2020.)

Zarzeka, A., Panczyk, M., Zmuda-Trzebiatowska, H., et al. (2017). Nurse prescribing, knowledge and attitudes of Polish nurses in the eve of extending their professional competencies: Cross-sectional study. *Acta Polioniae Pharmaceutica – Drug Research, 74*(3), 1031–1038.

Managing Difficult and Complex Patient Interactions

6

Donna L. Poole

This chapter coaches advanced practice registered nurses (Aprns) to deal with difficult and often complex clinical interactions that are inherent in professional practice and often related to prescribing. The basic tenet is that these are not "problem patients" but situations for which the APRN needs more knowledge, skill, and insight from self-reflection. Information that helps APRNs better understand why these difficult interactions develop and how they can impact patient-centered care is presented. Specific strategies to identify difficult interactions, respond to them appropriately, and build competence as a supportive and courageous APRN prescriber are discussed.

A hallmark of advanced practice registered nurse (APRN) practice is the expertise to establish caring, supportive relationships with patients in order to "make a difference" in patients' lives. Many APRNs attribute their work satisfaction and longevity in the role to these rewarding or inspiring relationships with patients (Stokowski et al., 2019).

At the same time, interactions with patients can be a source of significant stress. APRNs are often faced with clinical situations that are prompted by uncomfortable patient interactions that they find difficult or for which they feel ill prepared. There is usually little education offered to increase knowledge and skills and assist APRNs to manage these types of complex clinical interactions. Certain patient behaviors can be particularly uncomfortable for many clinicians. Common complex interactions may include:

- Substance-related concerns
- Boundary violations
- Behavioral health problems
- Unresolved or undiagnosed medical concerns
- Requests for inappropriate or unnecessary care including medications
- Not accepting recommended care.

The Advanced Practice Registered Nurse as a Prescriber, Second Edition. Edited by Louise Kaplan and Marie Annette Brown.
© 2021 John Wiley & Sons Ltd. Published 2021 by John Wiley & Sons Ltd.

In many complex clinical situations both the patient and the provider suffer. The word *patient* originally meant "one who suffers" and is derived from the Latin word *patiens*, meaning "I am suffering" (Merriam Webster, 2020). Commonly, difficult interactions leave the provider with feelings of psychological distress or a sense of failure. When a practitioner feels frustrated, uncertain, angry, manipulated, or controlled, the patient may be labeled a "problem patient."

Miksanek (2008) acknowledges the very human initial reactions that many providers experience with these interpersonal difficulties.

> Let's be blunt. It's hard to care for difficult patients. It's sometimes impossible to actually like them. This species of sick individuals tends to strain time, patience and resources. They often generate a cascade of phone calls. They sometimes demand a heap of medically unnecessary tests. They occasionally refuse recommended treatment. Many have unreasonable expectations. Some whine and gripe incessantly. A few threaten to sue. Almost all of them need at least thirty minutes – and want sixty minutes – of face time. . . . In their own unique ways, they make my professional life tricky. Even in my private life, they invade my thoughts – with disappointment, irritation and worry. (p. 1422)

While it may be assumed the patient is a difficult person with whom to interact, provider and healthcare system factors contribute to the situations (Moukaddam et al., 2017). Providers tend to blame patients for the difficult interactions; patients tend to blame the provider. Either can intervene to change the nature of the interaction; the provider wields the most influence and has the best opportunity to repair the interaction. Often a thoughtful and informed approach can prevent escalation of the current problematic interaction.

The concept of the "difficult patient" was first described from the physician's viewpoint in the 1970s. While nurses and other healthcare professionals have not as specifically conceptualized the "difficult patient" in the literature, discussions about conflict with patients are common (Cerit et al., 2020). The current emphasis on patient-centered care provides the opportunity to shift the focus of this concept to difficult or complex *interactions* so that more productive responses and targeted interventions can be developed.

Difficult interactions can be instigated by patients, providers, or the system in which the patient and provider meet (e.g. wait times, formulary restrictions). Strategies to handle the most common difficult situations may increase the practitioner's comfort and competence in managing difficult interactions, decrease work stress, and increase job satisfaction. This chapter provides a conceptual framework and strategies for managing some of the most common challenges APRNs may confront in their relationships with patients, particularly when prescribing.

KNOWLEDGE OF SELF AS THE FOUNDATION FOR PROFESSIONAL GROWTH

Knowledge of self is gained using multiple strategies which include self-awareness, mindfulness, and reflective practice. These strategies are interrelated and form the foundation of knowledge of self. Effective communication requires self-awareness that allows us to be conscious of our own views, ideals, wants, and needs, and how they differ from others. As we learn more about our personal beliefs and values, we can engage in objective self-examination to explore our own biases and positions, monitor our thoughts and feelings, and guide us to helpful and affirming actions. This is an important tool in the development of therapeutic relationships with patients. Self-awareness is one of the key components of emotional intelligence: the capacity to identify, express, evaluate, and instinctively self-regulate emotions (Schub & Smith, 2017).

Patient interactions are often considered to be difficult because of the intensity of feelings that may occur and unconscious feelings that may be inappropriate to the content and context of the relationship. Lack of conscious awareness can lead to challenges engaging with the patient such as difficulty empathizing; feelings of anger or impatience; recurrent anxiety, unease, or guilt; violations of boundaries; and behaviors that cannot be justified as therapeutic (Stuart, 2009).

Conscious awareness is required if the APRN is to accurately observe and productively engage the patient. One way to improve awareness is through Mindful Practice, which can be described as: "Clinicians' capacity for reflection, self-monitoring, and self-awareness during actual clinical practice in order to practice with clarity, insight, expertise, and compassion" (Epstein, 2020, p. 61). The components of mindfulness include self-awareness, self-regulation, and self-transcendence (Vago & Silbersweig, 2012).

Characteristics of mindfulness include attentiveness, curiosity, and presence. Attentiveness refers to awareness of external as well as internal data, biases, and cognitive deceptions that interfere with clinical decision making. Curiosity can create a communication opening in tense situations. Platt and Gordon (2004) advise "get curious, not furious" when interactions provoke anger in the provider. Presence is a purposeful practice of awareness, focus, and attention with the intent to understand and connect with patients (Brown-Johnson et al., 2019). The APRN may foster presence in a clinical encounter in a variety of ways:

- Prepare with intention (prepare and focus before greeting the patient)
- Listen intently and completely (sit down, lean forward, avoid interruptions)
- Agree on what matters most (incorporate patient priorities into the visit agenda)
- Connect with the patient's story (contemplate the life circumstances and influences on a patient's health, acknowledge efforts, and celebrate successes)
- Explore emotional cues (realize, name, and confirm the patient's emotions) (Zulman et al., 2020).

Mindfulness has benefits beyond that of improving interactions with patient. One study found a reduction in emotional difficulty, anxiety, and perceived stress in comparison to those who did not receive mindfulness training (Barattucci et al., 2019). APRNs with less perceived stress and anxiety are in the best position to successfully engage with patients of all perceived levels of difficulty. See Box 6.1.

Peplau (1951), a nursing pioneer in challenging interpersonal relationships, emphasized that in order to assist patients to meet their needs, the nurse must be aware of his or her own needs. Self-reflection is an important skill to help APRNs remain vigilant about their behavior and address areas

---

Box 6.1 Developing mindfulness in everyday practice

- Attempt to see a familiar situation with new eyes ("beginner's mind")
- Priming – create the expectation for mindfulness:
  - Pause or take a breath before entering the patient's room
  - Develop a habit or ritual, e.g. touch the doorknob of the exam room
  - Look at the patient rather than at the chart or screen
  - Create a "mantra" for daily practice, e.g. "it might not be so"
  - Find a moment of stillness in everyday practice
- Ask oneself reflective questions

Source: Epstein, 2020.

Box 6.2 Framework to guide reflective practice

What? This is the descriptive phase (all questions start with what)	So what? This is the theoretical/conceptual phase	Now what? At this phase we think about other ways of thinking or acting and choose the most appropriate
• What happened? • What did I do? • What did others do? • What did I feel? • What was I trying to achieve?	• So what is the importance of this? • So what is the significance for me? • So what more do I need to know about this? • So what have I learned about this?	• Now what should I do? • Now what would be the best thing to do? • Now what will I do? • Now what might be the consequences of this action?

Source: Based on Fyers & Greenwood, 2016.

---

of concern. It can also be useful for APRNs to focus on their emotional well-being to ascertain if a "need to be liked" and accepted by patients contributes to a conflict-avoidant approach to patient interactions.

There are several models used to teach Reflective Practice. The process takes time and develops with perseverance, but it can be as simple as asking "What?" "So what?" and "Now what?" (Box 6.2).

Reflective journaling is another widely available model that can be a fruitful pathway to cultivate insight. It can be used solely for personal use or as part of a more formal professional learning process. One model to develop critical reflection in journaling is the LEAP Guidelines: LEAP = "Learning from your Experiences as A Professional" (Litzelman et al., 2020). Beginners are taught to use a SOAP-like format, where S is the subjective experience, O is the objective data about the event, A is the assessment of causes of the event, and P the possible learning points.

When APRNs are faced with patient interactions that are highly charged and emotionally intense, reflective practices whether in group discussion or written, whether internally reviewed or reviewed with a mentor can lead to improvement in self-awareness.

Box 6.3 Case example of miscommunication

An APRN increasingly struggled with her primary care patient about specific brand medication requests that the patient said were learned about on TV. On her initial visit the patient asked for antibiotics for a cough and cold. On the next visit she requested Lunesta® for sleep problems. Subsequent visits over the next two years included requests for Soma® for neck pain, Xanax® for marital problems, Adderall® for fatigue, and a supply of antibiotics to have on hand for when she had sinus congestion infections. The APRN became increasingly frustrated during patient visits and asked the medical assistants to assist her with limiting the patient's visit time. When the patient sought care for abdominal discomfort, bloating, and weight gain, the APRN provided the patient with multiple educational handouts and links to websites. These addressed possible treatment approaches for irritable bowel syndrome and constipation. After six months the patient reported increasing discomfort and fatigue so the APRN ordered a pelvic ultrasound. This test revealed an ovarian mass that was diagnosed as advanced cancer. The family sued the APRN.

Why is it so important to develop introspection? Why are difficult patient interactions an excellent "pink flag" that indicates it is time for self-reflection and growth? APRNs can take advantage of their discomfort as a motivational prompt to learn something about oneself as a person and to develop new professional skills that could lessen discomfort. At the same time, these expanded negotiation and conflict resolution skills can be a protective factor to enhance safe practice. When we identify patients as difficult, our frustration could increase the risk that we may miss an important diagnostic cue or overlook a warning symptom.

The scenario in Box 6.3 highlights how the APRN's frustration with the patient's demands prompted her to spend less time with the patient, view the patient's symptoms in a more skeptical way, delay her usual assessment approaches, and thereby miss what could have been a more timely diagnosis. If the APRN had instead used her discomfort to motivate her to develop new skills to handle controversial medication requests, her avoidance could have been replaced by a new sense of capability.

MOTIVATIONAL INTERVIEWING AS THE FOUNDATION
FOR COUNSELING ABOUT CHANGE

Ineffective or inadequate communication is the root cause of nurse to nurse and nurse to patient/family stress (Bershad, 2019). Open, respectful, and compassionate communication, such as that exemplified by motivational interviewing (MI), can enhance APRN communication effectiveness.

MI was originally developed by William R. Miller and Stephen Rollnick in the 1980s to assist people with substance use disorders (Moyers, 2004). It is an evidence-based counseling approach that healthcare providers can use to help patients adhere to treatment recommendations. They observed that the more one tried to insert information and advice into others, the more people tended to back off and resist. Put simply, this approach posits that the provider and the patient can come together for a common goal when the provider asks the patient to describe why and how they might change for themselves. It is a clinical approach that helps people with mental health and substance use disorders and other chronic conditions such as diabetes, cardiovascular conditions, and asthma make positive behavioral changes to support better health. It is not simply a technique; rather it is a radical change in the approach to the patient from simply providing expert advice. It requires APRNs to understand more deeply that usually education alone to change behavior is much less effective.

MI incorporates an approach of shared decision making and the belief that the patient, like the customer, is always right. MI acknowledges that the patient is at the center of care and the health care provider must be respectful of and responsive to the individual patient's preferences, needs, and values. With MI, the patient's values guide all the clinical decision making. The APRN who employs MI is well positioned to assist the patient to explore ambivalence about change.

The spirit of MI is all about "coming alongside" the patient. The APRN listens deeply to the patient and demonstrates that they are heard and understood. The APRN can convey an understanding of what the patient feels without supporting an unhealthy behavior (Essenmacher, 2019).

The overall spirit of MI is described as **Collaborative, Evocative,** and **Honoring** of the patient's autonomy. There are four associated guiding principles of MI which can be remembered by the acronym RULE (Resist, Understand, Listen, and Empower):

- Resist the righting reflex
- Understand your patient's motivations
- Listen to your patient
- Empower your patient.
  (Rollnick et al., 2008)

One simple framework to implement MI is codified by the acronym OARS, which stands for **O**pen-ended questions, **A**ffirmation, **R**eflective listening, and **S**ummarize & teach back. See Box 6.4.

The goal to assist patients as they identify their own motivations for change and their own strategies to achieve those goals can help the APRN avoid frustration about different or conflicting goals. This congruence likely results in fewer difficult interactions and demonstrates that the APRN has respect and confidence in the power of the patient.

ETHICAL CONSIDERATIONS WHEN DEALING WITH DIFFICULT AND COMPLEX PATIENT INTERACTIONS

National Gallup polls in the United States repeatedly identify nurses as the public's most trusted profession (Reinhart, 2020). The professional ethics of APRNs have contributed to the public's esteem. Nonetheless, the complexity of prescribing and factors such as direct-to-consumer advertising of medication may create difficult clinical situations between APRNs and patients. When this occurs, the Code of Ethics for Nurses with Interpretive Statements (American Nurses Association [ANA], 2015) can provide guidance.

Box 6.4 OARS

O: Typically starts with who, what, when, or where questions. "Why" questions require more finesse as they can often come across as judgmental.

- Instead of: "Why didn't you take your medicine?" Try: "What was difficult about taking the medicine?"
- Instead of: "Why did you want that prescription?" Try: "Why is this medication important to you?"

A: Listen for recall, and restate examples of good decision making:

- "I think that's a great idea you have to use a medicine box."
- "I agree with your idea to change your diet before starting medication for high cholesterol."

R: Therapeutic conversations are made up of listening as well as questions. Listening can sometimes be the most difficult part of MI. Listen with purpose and pay attention to your intuition to pull out the important parts of a conversation. Reflective listening can be as simple as turning a question into a statement.

- Instead of: "Are you upset?" Try: "I sense that you are feeling upset about this."
- Review and rephrase a patient statement:
  - Patient: "Taking antidepressants always makes me nauseous."
  - APRN: "It sounds like you think that medication will make you feel worse."

S: Summarize any strengths that the patient has revealed as well as any action steps that have been considered. Consider asking the patient to repeat any instructions that have been provided in order to reinforce important learning.

- "So, you are going to put your electronic skills to work by setting an alarm on your phone to remind you to take your blood pressure medicine."
- "To make sure I've done my job, explain to me how you are going to monitor the effectiveness of your medication for diabetes."

Source: Modified from Bershad, 2019.

The first official Code of Ethics for Nurses was adopted by the ANA in 1950, with the current version adopted in 2015. While every aspect of the Code is relevant, the first, second, and fifth provisions are most applicable to dealing with complex patient interactions.

- **Provision 1**: The nurse practices with compassion and respect for the inherent dignity, worth, and unique attributes of every person.
- **Provision 2**: The nurse's primary commitment is to the patient, whether an individual, family, group, community, or population.
- **Provision 5**: The nurse owes the same duties to self as to others, including the responsibility to promote health and safety, preserve wholeness of character and integrity, maintain competence, and continue personal and professional growth. (ANA, 2015).

Provision 1 represents the core values and responsibilities of the profession. Most of the time, most nurses practice in a highly ethical manner and demonstrate respect for all their patients. However, this respect is more difficult to access when patients bring challenges to the patient–provider relationship that may lead to feelings of anxiety or discomfort. In these situations APRNs need to be particularly mindful to maintain a professional relationship without bias or prejudice. The Code of Ethics mandates that patients deserve respect, care, and the promotion of health and wellness even when the ARPN does not agree with the lifestyle, personal, or healthcare choices made by the patient. For example, a patient with opioid use disorder should not be judged or stigmatized. At the same time, the APRN has a professional obligation to address behavior that may be harmful to the patient yet maintain compassion and respect. This balanced approach can be difficult for many healthcare professionals and prompts them to seek additional skill development. Skills in MI are particularly relevant in these situations and can help determine the person's readiness for options such as medication assisted treatment or harm reduction approaches.

Over time, nursing has been acknowledged as a profession dedicated to caring for the underserved, social justice, and acceptance of others. For example, in the 1890s Lillian Wald created public health nursing and the Henry Street clinic to serve the poor immigrant community in the tenements of New York City (Encyclopedia Britannica, 2020). Nursing's history of ethical concern and activities on behalf of and for persons of color was apparent even before the 1960s civil rights movement (ANA, 2015). Consequently, our profession has a solid base to embrace the recent societal examination of institutional racism and to dedicate ourselves to the next step and actively support antiracist policy. According to Fowler, "patient personal attributes, circumstances, or life choices are never grounds for prejudice and may be used only to individualize care in accord with patient needs" (ANA, 2015, p. 12).

Provision 2 centers on the patient as the first loyalty of the nurse and on the primacy of the patient's interests. The APRN also has allegiance to self and family, an employer, and coworkers while the interests of the patient surpass the loyalties within the professional realm. If an APRN believes a patient's health would be improved with medication, and the patient is concerned about cost or side effects, shared decision making may allow the APRN to fulfill his or her professional duty to self and to the patient.

Provision 5 reflects the historical position that the nurse owes the same duty to self as to others. The notion of duty to self comes from the concept of universal obligations: if an obligation applies to everyone, then it must apply to the self. This includes the APRN caring for one's own health and physical and emotional well-being. Ultimately, the health and welfare of self and family may be expected to predominate. For example, in an emergency, an APRN would not be expected to put a patient above the health and welfare of self and family. At the same time, possible risks to the nurse's health and welfare need nuanced consideration to distinguish them from convenience and preference. While ethical considerations are a strong foundation, it is still essential for the APRN to seek support, whether it be educational, mentoring, or counseling, to prepare oneself for managing difficult patient interactions.

ENGAGING PATIENTS WITH SUBSTANCE-RELATED CONCERNS

The National Institute on Drug Abuse (NIDA) reports that the use of tobacco, alcohol, prescription drug misuse, and illicit drugs costs the United States $740 billion each year in expenses related to crime, lost work productivity, and healthcare (NIDA, 2020a). Misuse is defined as taking a prescription medication in a manner or dose other than prescribed. In 2016, more than 84 percent of all Americans had contact with a healthcare professional (NIDA, 2012, 2020b). Consequently, APRNs are positioned to identify and address complex clinical situations in which patients suffer from substance use disorders.

Evidenced-based screening tools for the non-medical use of prescription drugs are an important part of routine healthcare visits. SBIRT (Screening, Brief Intervention, and Referral to Treatment [Substance Abuse and Mental Health Services Administration, n.d.]) and NIDA Quick Screen (NIDA, 2012) are two resources in the public domain. Research indicates that a single question can be used to identify non-medical use of prescription drugs: "How many times in the past year have you used an illegal drug or used a prescription medication for non-medical reasons?" (Smith et al., 2010, p. 1156). Providers are sometimes reluctant to screen because they fear a positive response and have not yet developed the skills to respond appropriately. However, in a short conversation, the APRN can let patients know if and how their drug use may be putting their health at risk. The Five As of Intervention (Agency for Healthcare Research and Quality [AHRQ], 2012), was initially developed to help providers assist patients with smoking cessation. It has been adapted for use in managing other healthcare problems (Vallis et al., 2013), and it provides a structured framework for the APRN to use regardless of the substance or chronic healthcare problem. See Box 6.5.

The opioid epidemic in the United States has resulted in national and state guidelines to limit opioid prescribing. Some APRNs have concerns that prescribing opioids and other controlled substances such as benzodiazepines could contribute to the prevalence of substance use disorders. The prevention and reduction of prescription drug use disorders is an important consideration

---

Box 6.5 Five major steps to intervention (the "5 As")

- ASK – Use a formal screen or ask several questions related to substance use.
- ADVISE – If clinically indicated, in a clear, strong, and personalized manner advise the patient to make a change. This might be abstinence or other suggestions to reduce risky behavior.
- ASSESS – Determine the patient's willingness to make a change. Accept and acknowledge decisions not to change. Welcoming the conversation over time without judgement keeps the relationship going for discussions on another day.
- ASSIST – Brief counseling (MI, raising awareness, providing education) or pharmacotherapy for tobacco, alcohol, and opiates is available.
- ARRANGE – Set up follow-up appointments or refer to specialty care if needed. For integrated practices, this might include a "warm handoff" to a behavioral health or substance use disorder professional.

Source: Modified from AHRQ, 2012.

in patient care. However, to avoid controlled substances when they are needed because of that fear can decrease the quality of care delivered by APRNs. To successfully navigate between the dichotomy of relieving suffering and contributing to harm, it is important for the prescriber to develop expertise in talking to patients about their substance use.

Neuroscience continues to support the concept of addiction as a brain disease (NIDA, 2016). Some still question this etiology and culturally it has been viewed as a life choice at best, or more pejoratively as a moral failing (Heather, 2017). When patients experience socially discrediting stigmatization, they often develop internalized stigma that can prevent them from seeking and accepting medical treatment. Internalized stigma can lead to patient defense mechanisms, such as denial, in which they deny substance use even when presented with objective evidence such as a clinically verified urine drug screen or a breathalyzer (Kelly, 2018). The APRN who presents with a non-judgmental empathetic approach is in a much better position to have an honest, fruitful discussion with a patient about substance use. Non-stigmatizing language is also helpful to break down barriers. See Box 6.6.

THE OPIOID EPIDEMIC AS A PROMPT FOR DIFFICULT CONVERSATIONS

The United States is facing an epidemic of non-medical use of opioids, leading to over 46,000 deaths in 2018 from both prescription and illegal opioids (Wilson et al., 2020). At the same time, untreated pain remains a critical problem in our healthcare system. Chronic pain is estimated to affect 20% (50 million) of the US adult population, and 19.6 million (8%) US adults have "high-impact" chronic pain that limits life or work activities (Dahlhamer et al., 2018). These two public health crises require full attention by all clinicians. The relationship of the opioid crisis and prevalence of chronic pain creates an extremely complex healthcare problem, for which APRNs are well positioned to intervene.

Fueled by the opioid epidemic, the Comprehensive Addiction and Recovery Act of 2016 (CARA) amended the Controlled Substances Act and authorized nurse practitioners (NPs) for five years to fulfill the requirements to prescribe buprenorphine for addiction treatment (CADCA, 2016). Passage of the Substance Use-Disorder Prevention that Promotes Opioid Recovery and Treatment for Patients and Communities Act (SUPPORT) in 2018 also amended the Controlled Substances Act and permanently authorized NPs. The law authorized nurse anesthetists and nurse midwives for five years to prescribe buprenorphine for opioid use disorder (OUD).

Although the number of buprenorphine providers has increased, a treatment gap still exists in the care of patients with OUD. Ninety percent of waivered practitioners remain in urban counties of the United States (Andrilla et al., 2018). One year after the implementation of CARA, more than half of all rural counties still lacked a buprenorphine provider. NPs and physician assistants accounted for the added treatment availability in 56 counties, 43 of which were rural (Andrilla et al., 2019).

There is a continued need for APRNs to treat patients with OUDs. The utilization of medications for OUD usually involves a long-term commitment for both the provider and the patient. Inherent in the success of treatment is the

Box 6.6 Recovery Research Institute "Addictionary" – stigma alert

Potentially stigmatizing word/ expression	Suggested word/expression
Abuser	"A person with or suffering from addiction or substance use disorder"
Addict	"A person with or suffering from addiction or substance use disorder"
Alcoholic	"A person with or suffering from an alcohol use disorder"
Clean vs. dirty urine drug screens	"Positive" vs. "negative" urine drug screens
Dope sick	"Suffering from withdrawal"
Drug	Distinguish between a "medication" and a "non-medically used psychoactive substance"
Dry drunk	"Individuals who no longer drink but continue to behave dysfunctionally"
Enabling	*Do not use; infers judgment and blame*
Lapse, relapse, or slip	"Resumed or experienced a recurrence of substance use"
Opioid replacement therapy (ORT)	"Opioid substitution therapy" or "opioid maintenance therapy"
Medication assisted treatment (MAT)	"Medications for addiction treatment"
Prescription drug misuse	"Non-medical use of a psychoactive substance"

Source: Modified from Addictionary – Glossary of Substance Use Disorder Terminology, Recovery Research Institute, n.d. https://www.recoveryanswers.org/addiction-ary/ (accessed 7 September 2020).

acceptance that OUD, and all substance use disorders, are brain diseases, not moral failings. Moreover, it is imperative to develop the perspective that OUD is a chronic disease that can be managed in a primary care context. APRNs can have a tremendous impact to lessen the burden of substance use when they provide access to treatment for patients with OUD, particularly in rural and underserved areas. Medications for addiction treatment improve the quality of life for patients with OUD, support their return to work, and reduce comorbidities. Most importantly, they save lives (Moore, 2019).

APRNs can make a significant difference in the life of individuals with substance use issues in multiple ways, if they develop the skills necessary to have difficult conversations. They can assist patients to enter treatment with the goal of recovery and engage patients in harm reduction to sustain life. Most importantly, APRNs help patients restore their dignity and serve as powerful role models for colleagues when they treat patients with kindness and respect. The approach taken by the APRN can either help or hinder the patient's recovery, as so eloquently explained by Dr Kimberly Sue, medical director of the Harm Reduction Coalition.

I feel strongly that practicing clinicians often disregard the dignity, autonomy, and well-being of people who use drugs – to the point that what clinicians say and do can actually increase harm and increase death. Whether you're a generalist or whether you're taking care of people with substance use, be nice to people who use drugs and understand that they come with long histories of trauma and disrespect at the hands of health care providers. That's something that I've learned being in the trenches with people who use drugs, who are cast into the shadows and the alleys. (Sue, 2020, p. 6.)

MANAGING INTERACTIONS THAT CAN LEAD TO BOUNDARY VIOLATIONS

Boundaries are the basis of all human relationships and begin with an infant's initial awareness about "me" versus "my caregivers." In the healthcare relationship, boundaries help determine what the patient and the APRN will each bring to the encounter. Usually there are limits to what occurs in the therapeutic relationship, but this is often unspoken. It includes implicit agreement about the roles each will play, how they will speak to each other, and the agenda for the visit (Platt & Gordon, 2004). Many difficult interactions are based upon conflicting expectations between the patient and the APRN (Box 6.7). When there is confusion over the role of the APRN there is a potential for stressful interactions.

According to the National Council of State Boards of Nursing, "Professional boundaries are the spaces between the nurse's power and the patient's vulnerability" (NCSBN, 2018). There is an inherent power differential between the patient and the APRN. The APRN is aware of the personal and medical history of the patient. In addition to intimate knowledge about the patient, the APRN often has examined the physical body of the patient. Because of this imbalance of information, the APRN must be aware and respectful of the power imbalance. Necessarily, the therapeutic relationship must be patient centered.

Boundary "crossings" are brief excursions across the professional lines of behavior that may be inadvertent, well intended, or even purposeful with therapeutic intent (NCSBN, 2018). For example, the APRN who shares too much personal information crosses a boundary. When the APRN talks more about the self than the patient, there is the potential for adverse consequences. Fortunately, when recognized it is possible to return to established boundaries. An example

---

Box 6.7 Case example: expectations

A primary care APRN met with a new patient for the first time. The patient had moved from another state and had the expectation that her medications from her previous provider would be continued. Included in the medication list was a stimulant that was being prescribed off label for depression. The APRN agreed to continue all other medications, as they seemed appropriate, but declined to continue the off-label stimulant at that first appointment. The enraged patient left the practice vowing never to return and filed a complaint with the state board of nursing against the APRN for abandonment. After investigation, the case was closed as "No Violation" but the reviewers felt the APRN may have prevented some anguish on the part of the patient and the APRN if expectations and a plan for further action had been developed in concert with the patient.

of a therapeutic crossing may be when the APRN gives the patient a small token gift meant as inspiration towards a health goal. Repeated boundary crossings are discouraged.

Behavior tends to occur on a continuum rather than always being right or wrong. For any given situation, the facts need to be reviewed to determine whether there was a boundary crossing or violation. Questions to ask during this review include:

- What was the intent of the boundary crossing?
- Was it for a therapeutic purpose?
- Was it in the patient's best interest?
- Did it optimize or detract from the care of the patient?
- Did the APRN consult with a supervisor or colleague? (NCSBN, 2018).

Boundaries can be a highly charged issue as the APRN makes decisions about social media. Because of numerous privacy violations and problems, some agencies, schools, and healthcare institutions have developed guidelines about how employees will or will not engage with patients. Should the APRN and patient ever be "friends" on social media? This can be a particularly difficult question to address in small, insular communities. As social media becomes even more ubiquitous, APRNs will be faced with decisions on a regular basis about whether or not to blur the lines between professional and personal lives.

An extreme form of boundary violation is professional sexual misconduct. This includes any behavior that is seductive, sexually demeaning, harassing, or reasonably interpreted as sexual by the patient. Professional sexual misconduct violates the trust of the relationship and is an extremely serious violation of the nurse's professional responsibility to a patient (NCSBN, 2014).

Typically, boundary crossings or violations may be part of a larger set of issues related to professional behavior. Some individuals are more prone to boundary violations than others. Additionally, there are warning signs or "red flag" behaviors that can trigger the APRN to examine one's own and/or colleagues' professional–patient interactions (Box 6.8).

APRNs without self-knowledge and insight are at greater risk for boundary violations. It is complex and difficult to discern what makes one healthcare professional act on sexual feelings and another not. Depression, failed relationships, and other traumas can increase the vulnerability of the APRN (Indiana State Nurses Association, 2019).

If a patient crosses professional boundaries such as being sexually provocative, it is important to address this in a timely, direct, and highly sensitive way. Outright rejection of the patient or their advances may lead to false accusations. Careful documentation and collegial support can be a particularly critical part of the process of self-protection. Possible approaches include: leave the room and return with another professional; document the actions taken in the medical record; keep a log of calls and contacts by the patient; and keep the originals of any correspondence or gifts in case they are needed as evidence (Finnegan, 2016).

Box 6.8 Red flag behaviors

- Discussing intimate or personal issues with a patient
- Engaging in behaviors that could reasonably be interpreted as flirting
- Keeping secrets with a patient or for a patient
- Believing that you are the only one who truly understands or can help the patient
- Spending more time than is necessary with a particular patient
- Speaking poorly about colleagues or your employment setting with the patient and/ or family
- Showing favoritism
- Meeting a patient in settings besides those used to provide direct patient care or when you are not a work

Source: NCSBN, 2018.

ENGAGING PATIENTS WITH BEHAVIORAL HEALTH ISSUES

This section addresses several patient behavioral health issues that may contribute to difficult, complex interactions across multiple providers and include patients with borderline personality disorder (BPD), intensive health anxiety, and somatic disorders. When APRNs have more in-depth information about these important mental issues, they may be able to tailor their approaches and comments in a way to avoid difficult conversations. APRNs in psychiatric nursing often declare that "every nurse is a mental health nurse." Given that about three-quarters of all patients on a primary care provider's daily clinical schedule will have a behavioral component (Sherman et al., 2017), it would be hard to argue against the assertion. Because of the stigma towards mental illness in our society, it is not surprising that many patients seek care for psychological issues from their primary care providers. While integrated primary care and behavioral healthcare practices are increasingly common, APRNs in primary care and nurse midwives caring for women in the perinatal period must be prepared to manage behavioral health issues independently. Often patients will refuse referrals to behavioral health providers, even when they are available in the community. This may be due to concerns about stigma or financial concerns related to higher co-pays or more out-of-pocket expenses.

Borderline personality disorder

Patients who meet the criteria for BPD are often thought to be "difficult." Numerous studies have correlated characteristics of BPD with characteristics of difficult patients, and at least one scholar has argued that the category of "borderline" was created to label patients who are perceived to be difficult (Sulzer, 2015). Sulzer contends that patients with BPD are often viewed as "morally suspect people" and that many providers feel as if patients with BPD should not be patients at all. In her study, she found that many providers preferred to care for people with schizophrenia who were considered to have a "biological sickness" rather people with BPD who were considered to have a "moral badness" rather than sickness. Sulzer terms this the "demedicalization" which is replaced with the stigmatization of patient care. This outcome of clinician beliefs can lead to patients with BPD being actively or passively denied care. This is perhaps most blatant in psychiatric practices where clinicians will actively state that they do not treat BPD. In primary care it is more likely to happen when the clinician takes an antagonistic approach to the patient who may then lose control. These patients are then discharged from the practice based upon their provoked bad behavior which is a hallmark of their illness.

The knowledgeable APRN will be able to recognize BPD and provide appropriate treatment to patients in a way that can minimize frustration and maximize satisfaction. This expertise is particularly important since it is believed that prevalence of patients with BPD is four to five times higher in primary care than in the general population (Wlodarczyk et al., 2018). Common clinical presentations include:

- History of "provider shopping"
- Legal suits against healthcare professionals
- Suicide attempts
- Several brief marriages or unsuccessful intimate relationships
- Idealization of the APRN as the "most wonderful" provider compared to others
- Excessive interest in the APRN's personal life
- Attempts to test or invade professional boundaries (Wehbe-Alamah & Wolgamott, 2014).

A few simple strategies can assist the APRN to maintain professional deportment that will allow the APRN to provide appropriate care for the patient with BPD. Some strategies include:

- Set clear boundaries on the role of the APRN (see section on boundary violations in this chapter)
- Schedule regular appointments for check-ins and to avoid crisis appointments
- Develop a crisis management plan in concert with the patient for anticipated problems that may lead to emergency department visits
- De-escalate emotionally intense confrontations with a calm and neutral demeanor
- Coordinate and collaborate with other involved providers to avoid the process of devaluation-idealization between providers (often referred to as "splitting").

SOMATIC SYMPTOMS AND RELATED DISORDERS
Patients with extreme health anxiety

Patients who present with physical symptoms or complaints for which there is no obvious medical morbidity may experience a somatic symptom or related disorder. Nevertheless, these patients have significant distress and impairment. Some patients may be highly anxious about a feared outcome, fueled in part by an understandable cause, such as when all family members have died of cancer. They are more commonly encountered in primary care and other medical settings and are less common in psychiatric and other mental health settings.

Many APRNs may not have been exposed to or educated about these diagnoses that are common across most practice settings. While patients who meet the full criteria for a specific diagnosis may be uncommon, it is estimated that up to 40% of primary care patients have medically unexplained symptoms (Raj, 2020). Conversations about unexplained symptoms with their potential for misunderstanding, frustration, and judgmental responses are often the first step in a difficult, complex patient interaction.

Recognition of somatic symptoms

Patients with somatic symptom disorders may not be immediately apparent, and the APRN may only begin to suspect this after a full work-up that may have included referrals to specialists. However, the initial work-up needs to be thorough and consistent with the APRN's usual approach to quality care. Patients with mental illness are more likely to have undetected organic pathological conditions because symptoms were ascribed to psychiatric symptoms rather than medical disease (Moukaddam et al., 2015).

When patients are distressed or impaired by their unexplained symptoms, the APRN needs to be particularly attentive and mindful to avoid potential conflict. Some patients are relieved when reassurance is provided, and other patients are even more distressed. They may feel that the APRN does not believe the suffering they are experiencing. APRNs are often frustrated and uncomfortable because they are unable to remedy the illness. Somatic disorders do not fit well within our acute illness model and are best thought of and approached as a chronic condition. The most important tools at this point are empathy and acceptance. Being empathetic toward the patient and perceptive of the suffering experienced is critical to maintaining an open relationship with the patient. The APRN must convey an understanding and acceptance of the patient's discomfort.

APRN: The tests have all come back negative and there is no serious disease that is causing your abdominal pain.

PATIENT: Then why do I have all this pain? Do you think I'm faking?

APRN: Not at all. I know that you are in a great deal of distress and have been suffering with this pain for a while.

PATIENT: Maybe they should do surgery just to check it out.

APRN: Surgery is risky and could give you more problems than you have now.

PATIENT: How about a strong pain pill?

APRN: I don't want to give you something that could have serious side effects and not solve the underlying cause of the pain.

PATIENT: I don't know how long I can take it.

APRN: It must be frustrating for you not to have an immediate solution. I want to see you regularly so that we can monitor the situation. Having pain, when the cause is not clear, can be incredibly stressful. Let's look at some other ways that we can manage your stress.

Somatic symptom disorders remain poorly understood and even current theoretical perspectives can be complex (Landa et al., 2012). It is essential, however, to avoid the separation of mind and body and instead utilize the current proliferation of holistic health approaches that support integrative etiologies of health problems. Likewise, the differentiation of "psychological" versus "organic" is not a fruitful path, since the patient's condition reflects both. The APRN can assist the patient to understand the symptom in socially acceptable terms such as muscle tension, stress, fatigue, or other common experiences. For most patients, a total alleviation of symptoms is not realistic. However, in addition to the supportive ARPN, there are other strategies that can assist with coping. For patients who are open to psychotherapy, cognitive behavioral therapy is particularly helpful. Further valuable options include: behavioral activation, problem solving, relaxation training, mindfulness, and meditation. All of these approaches include skills that can be taught and are supported by evidence (Moukaddam et al., 2015).

It is important to distinguish somatic symptom disorders from two related disorders, factitious disorder and malingering (American Psychiatric Association, 2013). A factitious disorder is the intentional production or feigning of physical or psychological signs or symptoms. The motivation for the behavior is to assume the sick role and obtain some specific rewards, e.g. sympathy and special attention. Malingering is the purposeful feigning of physical symptoms for external gain such as economic gain, avoiding legal responsibility, or improving physical well-being. Malingering is not considered to be a mental illness. In contrast, with somatic symptom disorders where there are no obvious gains or incentives for the patient, the physical symptoms are not willfully adopted or feigned.

Management of somatic symptoms

Patients with somatic symptom disorders may present the APRN with the common dilemma of addressing requests for an unwarranted medication. A key aspect of management is building a trusting, respectful relationship where a patient experiences the practitioner's caring and compassion. Discussion of the patient's suffering caused by this disorder is an important part of the therapeutic conversation. Discussions that include mental healthcare referrals as part of the treatment plan may then be more successful when the emphasis is on management of the patient's suffering concerning a symptom rather than implying the symptom is "not real" and therefore requires psychiatric care.

When a patient with somatic symptom disorder is resistant to a recommendation for mental health therapy, that resistance needs to be carefully explored. Sometimes it may be relatively straightforward to help the patient deal with the anxiety associated with the selection of a psychiatric, mental health APRN from a pool of unfamiliar, perhaps even intimidating healthcare professionals. At other times, the resistance may be intractable, and the patient does not desire to come to terms with a health situation, at least at this time. It is important though that APRNs utilize the approaches they usually employ with other patient treatment refusals. Many patients require multiple discussions about a management strategy and the APRN can remember the interpretation "not for now."

Patients with somatic symptoms may benefit from a structured approach to interactions with their primary and specialty care providers (see Box 6.9). Scheduled appointments demonstrate to the patient that the APRN takes his or

---

Box 6.9 Practice management strategies for somatic symptoms

- Recognize that patients may have physical symptoms for which there is no medical explanation, without malingering or feigning symptoms.
- Schedule regular, brief follow-up office visits with the patient.
  - Conduct a brief physical examination to provide comfort and reassurance.
  - Avoid unnecessary tests, surgeries, and referrals.
  - Prescribe medications with caution and only for specific indications.
  - Medications should be scheduled rather than as needed to avoid rewarding a symptom with a pill.
- Limit frequent telephone calls and "urgent" visits. Advise the patient to keep a list of concerns to discuss at the next regularly scheduled visit.
- Focus interventions on functioning and management of the disorder, not on diagnosis and cure. Issues to be addressed may include:
  - Stress reduction
  - Lifestyle modification
  - Meaning of the illness to the patient
- Include the patient's family in the development of the treatment plan if appropriate and possible.
- Treat comorbid physical and psychiatric disorders with appropriate interventions.

---

her concerns seriously. At the same time, regular rather than on-demand appointments may reduce provider reinforcement of the "sick" role among patients with somatic symptoms.

Regardless of the patient's openness to appropriate treatment, APRNs must set boundaries and discuss the rationale for limiting inappropriate medications or other treatments and instead emphasize how the patient's quality of care could be affected. It is important for APRNs to develop comfort and skill in dealing with requests for unnecessary care. Over-prescribing can expose the patient to potential health risks, utilization of financial resources, and increased demands on the healthcare system.

RESPONDING TO A REQUEST FOR INAPPROPRIATE TREATMENT

Direct-to-consumer advertising coupled with extensive health information on the Internet and media coverage of healthcare has changed the nature of interactions between APRNs and patients. Internet information, which is not always accurate or interpreted correctly, has prompted many patients to request a medication, diagnostic test, or treatment they have read about or seen in the media. Sometimes these requests are appropriate and other times they are not. Patients make inappropriate requests for a variety of reasons and motivations. Many patients legitimately believe these requests are in their best interest and believe the convincing case presented on TV. Consequently they do not understand why the APRN does not agree. APRNs, in contrast, do not want to seem cold, uncaring, or withholding of appropriate treatments. There is little in the literature to guide APRNs on how to respond empathetically and to "just say no."

First, consider whether the patient's medication request is appropriate. Seek to understand what they were thinking and/or feeling about the medication after they viewed the ad. Perhaps the advertisement on the newest allergy medication prompted your patient to realize that they could actually feel better if their allergies were well controlled. If, however, the request is truly inappropriate then it may help to say that you wish you could fulfill their request but you have a significant concern. An example of one approach to a difficult situation could be to discuss with the patient how acquiescence to their medication request which is not safe, effective, or appropriate could be viewed as malpractice by colleagues or health systems. Similarly, it may be useful to help the patient understand the new imperatives of the current healthcare arena such as evidence-based practice, clinical guidelines, professional organization recommendation, and institutional policy that guides or limits practitioners. Reinforcing the message that appropriate care is quality care can lead to greater patient satisfaction and is a particularly relevant foundation for prescribing medications (see Box 6.10). Speaking succinctly with authority with an evidence-based rationale is often met with a positive response. Patients may also respond well when they are convinced that the APRN has put the patient's interests first. Rather than setting a limit on the patient, place the limit on yourself: "I'm open to considering anything that would be safe and effective for you, but I could not allow myself to prescribe something that could cause more harm than good."

Online resources and printed materials can also be useful to review with patients. For example, a quite common request in primary and urgent care is for antibiotics to treat a viral respiratory infection. Education about the nature of viral illnesses often manages these requests. The Centers for Disease Control and Prevention (CDC) has developed resource materials for clinicians and

---

Box 6.10 Strategies to say no

Keep it simple: Provide a concise medical explanation at a level the patient can understand. Repeat if necessary, but do not provide extensive or defensive explanations.

Accept responsibility for the decision: This is your decision so do not disempower yourself by blaming an employer, the Drug Enforcement Administration, or some other authority. While it is appropriate to cite standards of practice, here again, a lengthy explanation is not warranted.

Understand why you are making the decision: If you do not have good rationale for the clinical decision you are making, it will be difficult to make it clear to the patient. However, there are those times when an expert APRN will be guided by experience and intuition. In these instances, it might be appropriate to buy time. Tell the patient you want to think about the request or seek consultation from a trusted colleague. Patients by and large appreciate that you do not want to do anything that might cause them harm.

Put the patient first: Telling patients there is an important reason not to prescribe or provide a treatment is generally effective.

Agree to disagree: There are times when a patient is willing to "take the risk" and is insistent upon their preferred mode of treatment. When an APRN reaches an impasse with a patient, it can be interpreted as a genuine disagreement. Suggest that you agree to disagree and underscore your respect for them and their point of view. However, let them know that you also have respect for yourself and will not do what you believe to be harmful to them or in your estimation is poor nursing practice.

patients that can be accessed on the CDC website (CDC, 2019a, 2019b). Their campaign called "Be Antibiotics Aware" was developed to help providers deal with the problem of antibiotic resistance. Increasingly, as evidence-based practice and research about the translation of evidence into practice take hold, there is a deepening awareness that saying no to patients often involves a difficult clinical conversation. Patient requests may cause an anxiety-provoking situation for some APRNs. However, listening carefully to the patient's intention followed by polite, firm, direct, and brief explanations with a clear decision generally provides greater satisfaction to both parties.

Many experienced practitioners were educated prior to this new evidence-oriented environment – many in a time when patients and practitioners worked with the understanding that "the provider knows best" and clinical experience was considered paramount. A new set of negotiation, collaboration, and conflict resolution skills is now an essential part of the APRN toolkit to manage the complex arena of prescribing medications, especially in this era of evidence-based practice.

PATIENT ISSUES ABOUT THEIR TREATMENT RECOMMENDATIONS

The decision not to accept healthcare provider recommendations about treatment by patients is more the norm than the exception. Data regarding patient adherence to medications are limited and there is no consensus as to what constitutes adequate adherence. Studies show that 20–30% of patients never fill their prescriptions (Shea, 2019). In addition to problematic follow-through with medications, resistance to recommendations regarding diet, exercise, sleep, alcohol use, and cessation of the use of tobacco products and other harmful substances commonly occurs. The best predictor of patient adherence is thought to be the quality of the therapeutic relationship and the experience of being heard and understood. Powerful factors can be the APRN's skillful listening, kindness, and compassion. A simple question *"How do you feel about taking this medicine?"* may influence whether the APRN even prescribes the medication.

While there are no individual characteristics that predict adherence, factors leading to non-adherence include:

- Poor explanations by APRNs
- Patient failure to understand the explanations
- Confusing written materials or materials beyond the patient's reading level
- Treatment cost in terms of time, money, comfort, or effort
- Concern about troublesome or dangerous side effects
- Lack of belief that the recommendations will be helpful
- Conflict between the patient, the patient's family, and the APRN's beliefs about illness
- Patient fatigue or forgetfulness
  (Platt & Gordon, 2004).

It can be difficult for a patient to do a risk–benefit analysis about a medication they have never taken. They may have little sense of the "future benefit" or how they may feel if a medication was effective. Without the ability to imagine feeling better, decision making can be clouded by anxiety about side effects or fear of the unknown. Some patients may have spiritual, religious, cultural, or family value systems that emphasize acceptance of all life circumstances that occur, and make medications unnecessary. Other patients approach their lives with an overall passivity or a hypersensitization to using medication from a family history of medication abuse. It can be unacceptable or unimaginable to some patients to try to envision health improvement through medication therapy. The APRN's core philosophy of patient-centered care can help prevent these situations from becoming difficult interactions.

The Choice Triad as an approach to address differences

Resistance to requests and recommendations occurs either when the patient does not do what the practitioner advises or when the provider does not do what the patient desires. Shea (2019) describes what he refers to as the "Choice Triad," which are the three criteria used by all healthcare professionals, nationally and internationally, when personally deciding whether to prescribe medications:

1. They [patients] feel there is something wrong with them from which they want relief.
2. They feel motivated to try a medication because they believe it has the potential to bring the relief from their perceived problem (or perhaps prevent a serious future problem as with a vaccine).
3. They believe that the benefits of taking the medication outweigh the risks.

When healthcare professionals use words such as resistance, non-compliance, or non-adherence, this conveys the opinion that the patient is not doing what the healthcare professional wanted. Shea proposes instead the term *medication interest* as the core concept in discussions with patients and suggests the Choice Triad as a framework to discuss medications with patients (Box 6.11).

It is important to first assess if the patient feels something is wrong. For example, a patient with schizophrenia who experiences anosognosia will likely not take a medication voluntarily. Many people with hypertension do not experience symptoms, do not understand or believe the possible consequences, or do not know someone who was untreated and had a stroke or heart attack. They may not view elevated blood pressure as a health threat. The patient who does not believe something is wrong will not want to take an antipsychotic that might induce tardive dyskinesia or metabolic syndrome. From the patient's point of view, these preferences are understandable.

The second tenet of the Choice Triad guides the APRN to identify what the patient wants (see Box 6.12). A discussion focused on the patient's hopes and dreams as well as their areas of discouragement can communicate caring. For example, the joy in relief from depression or hypertension may be dampened if the patient develops sexual dysfunction. They may value a satisfying sexual life as more important than a reduction in blood pressure, anxiety, or depression.

The third tenet of the Choice Triad relates to what patients may have to give up or experience to treat their disease. Patients are often willing to endure some discomfort such as mild, transient side effects from a medication if the situation

---

Box 6.11 The Choice Triad

1. Uncover the patient's views on current medications or the concept of taking medications at all:
   - "How do you feel about your current medications?"
   - "What are your feelings about taking medications in general?"
2. Introduce the clinician's personal approach as a prescriber to the use of medication:
   - "My goal as an APRN is to always give you the best advice."
   - "In my own life, I only take medications when I feel that I really need them and feel that the benefits outweigh the risks. I take the same approach with my patients."
   - "Together we want to find a medicine that you are genuinely interested in taking because it makes you feel better and/or is doing what you want it to do."
   - "I always try to fill my patients in on the side effects and the pros and cons of using medications."
3. Provide ample introduction to the pros & cons and collaboratively arrive at a decision to use a new medication.

Box 6.12 Case example: patient-centered care

A family nurse practitioner (FNP) was exploring the goals and ambitions held by a 36-year-old man with type 2 diabetes and hypertension. The FNP discovered that while she was focused on lowering the patient's blood glucose and blood pressure, the patient was not. Instead, his focus in life was a promotion at work, preparation for fatherhood, and purchasing a new home. This led to a productive discussion of ways to achieve his goals, none of which directly related to his medications. However, eventually he was able to identify how managing his medications better might assist him with progress toward his goals.

---

will improve. If not forewarned though, the patient may assume the medication has detrimental effects instead of improvement in his or her condition.

Patient-centered care can help providers and patients remain hopeful and connected to each other. If patients believe they need help, if they are consulted about the nature of the problem, and if they are included in the discussion of the risks and benefits, they are more likely to actively participate and engage in medication recommendations. Placing the patient at the center of the treatment plan creates a working alliance between the APRN and patient that limits the frustrations of both.

CONCLUSION

The important theme throughout this chapter is that there are "difficult situations" or "difficult interactions" rather than "difficult patients." Often, these are not flaws with the patient but rather situations in which the APRN simply lacks knowledge or skills to manage the situation. Through self-awareness, ethical treatment, and increased skill building, APRNs can learn to manage many of the common communication problems in the patient–nurse relationship.

Communication problems in healthcare may arise as providers put greater emphasis on diseases and their management, than on people, their lives, and their health problems. These concepts of holistic care are the quintessential hallmark of nursing and often are described as part of nursing's unique perspective about the value of prescriber–patient partnerships. As with all prescribers, APRN–patient interactions about medication are inherently vulnerable to all the challenges previously discussed. Even with the increased pace of practice today, APRNs can prioritize their communication with patients, especially surrounding prescribing, as a priority that cannot be compromised. Rewards are often evident if the APRN is able to establish strong connections with patients and thereby experience the deep satisfaction of "making a difference".

REFERENCES

Agency for Healthcare Research and Quality. (2012). *Five Major Steps to Intervention (The "5 A's")*. Rockville, MD: Agency for Healthcare Research and Quality.

American Nurses Association. (2015). *Code of Ethics for Nurses with Interpretive Statements*. Silver Springs, MD: ANA. Retrieved from https://www.nursingworld.org/practice-policy/nursing-excellence/ethics/code-of-ethics-for-nurses/coe-view-only/. (Accessed 7 September 2020.)

American Psychiatric Association. (2013). *Diagnostic and Statistical Manual of Mental Disorders, Fifth Edition*. Arlington, VA: American Psychiatric Association, p. 663.

Andrilla, C.H.A., Coulthard, C., & Patterson, D.G. (2018). Prescribing practices of rural physicians waivered to prescribe buprenorphine. *American Journal of Preventive Medicine, 54*(6 Suppl 3), S208–S214.

Andrilla, C.H.A., Moore, T.E., Patterson, D.G., & Larson, E.H. (2019). Geographic distribution of providers with a DEA waiver to prescribe buprenorphine for the treatment of opioid use disorder: A 5-year update. *Journal of Rural Health, 35*(1), 108–112.

Barattucci, M., Padovan, A.M., Vitale, E., et al. (2019). Mindfulness-based IARA model® proves effective to reduce stress and anxiety in health care professionals. A six-month follow-up study. *International Journal of Environmental Research and Public Health, 16*(22), 4421.

Bershad, D. (2019). Motivational interviewing: A communication best practice. *American Nurse Today, 14*(9), 96–98.

Brown-Johnson, C., Schwartz, R. Maitra, A., et al. (2019). What is clinician presence? A qualitative interview study comparing physician and non-physician insights about practices of human connection. *BMJ Open, 9*, e030831.

CADCA. (2016). Comprehensive Addiction and Recovery Act (CARA). Retrieved from https://www.cadca.org/comprehensive-addiction-and-recovery-act-cara. (Accessed 7 September 2020.)

Centers for Disease Control and Prevention. (2019a). Annual Surveillance Report of Drug-Related Risks and Outcomes – United States Surveillance

Special Report. Atlanta: Centers for Disease Control and Prevention, US Department of Health and Human Services.

Centers for Disease Control and Prevention. (2019b). Get smart: Know when antibiotics work. Atlanta: Centers for Disease Control and Prevention, US Department of Health and Human Services.

Cerit, K., Karatas, T., & Ekici, D. (2020). Behaviours of healthcare professionals towards difficult patients: A structural equation modelling study. *Nursing Ethics*, 27(2), 554–566.

Dahlhamer, J., Lucas, J., Zelaya, C., et al. (2018). Prevalence of chronic pain and high-impact chronic pain among adults – United States, 2016. *Morbidity and Mortality Weekly Report*, 67(36), 1001–1006.

Encyclopedia Britannica. (2020). Henry Street Settlement. Retrieved from https://www.britannica.com/topic/henry-street-settlement. (Accessed 7 September 2020.)

Epstein, R. (2020). Mindful practice. In M.D. Feldman & J.F. Christensen (Eds) *Behavioral medicine* (p. 61). New York: McGraw Hill.

Essenmacher, C. (2019). Quick tip for motivational interviewing. APNA *News: The Psychiatric Nursing Voice*, March 2019, Members Corner Edition.

Finnegan, J. (2016). When the tables turn and patients try to seduce doctors. Fierce Healthcare. Retrieved from https://fiercehealthcare.com/practices/when-tables-are-turned-and-patients-try-to-seduce-doctors. (Accessed 7 September 2020.)

Fyers, K., & Greenwood, S. (2016). Cultural safety: developing self-awareness through reflective practice. *Nursing Review*, 16(2), 28–29.

Heather, N. (2017). Q: Is addiction a brain disease or a moral failing? A: neither. *Neuroethics*, 10(1), 115–124.

Indiana State Nurses Association. (2019). Basics of professional boundaries and sexual misconduct for nurses. *ISNA Bulletin*, 45(1), 9–11.

Kelly, J.F. (2018). Helping patients with stigma and addiction. *The Carlat Addiction Treatment Report*, 6(1).

Landa, A., Peterson, B.S., & Fallon, B.A. (2012). Somatoform pain: A developmental theory and translational research review. *Psychosomatic Medicine*, 74(7), 717–727.

Litzelman, D.K., Dicorcia, M., Cotingham, A., & Inui, T.S. (2020). Teaching behavioral medicine: Theory & practice. In M.D. Feldman & J.F. Christensen (Eds) *Behavioral medicine* (p. 542). New York: McGraw Hill.

Merriam Webster. (2020). Patient. Retrieved from http://unabridged.merriam-webster.com. (Accessed 7 September 2020.)

Miksanek, T. (2008). On caring for "difficult" patients. *Health Affairs*, 27(5), 1422–1428.

Moore, D.J. (2019) Nurse practitioners' pivotal role in ending the opioid epidemic. *The Journal for Nurse Practitioners*, 15(5), 323–327.

Moukaddam, N., AufderHeide, E., Flores, A., & Tucci, V. (2015). Shift, interrupted: Strategies for managing difficult patients including those with personality disorders and somatic symptoms in the emergency department. *Emergency Medicine Clinics of North America*, 33, 797–810.

Moukaddam, N., Flores, A., Matorin, A, et al. (2017). Difficult patients in the emergency department. *Psychiatry Clinics of North America, 40*, 379–395.

Moyers, T.T. (2004). History and happenstance: How motivational interviewing got its start. *Journal of Cognitive Psychotherapy: An International Quarterly, 18*(4), 291–298.

National Council of State Boards of Nursing. (2014). Professional boundaries in nursing – video transcript. Chicago, IL: NCSBS.

National Council of State Boards of Nursing. (2018). A nurse's guide to professional boundaries. Chicago, IL: NCSBS.

National Institute on Drug Abuse. (2012). Resource guide: screening for drug use in general medical settings. Retrieved from https://www.drugabuse. gov/publications/resource-guide-screening-drug-use-in-general-medical-settings. (Accessed 7 September 2020.)

National Institute on Drug Abuse. (2016). Review article reinforces support for brain disease model of addiction. Retrieved from https://www.drugabuse. gov/news-events/news-releases/2016/01/review-article-reinforces-support-brain-disease-model-addiction. (Accessed 7 September 2020.)

National Institute on Drug Abuse. (2020a). Trends & statistics. Retrieved from https://www.drugabuse.gov/related-topics/trends-statistics. (Accessed 7 Sepetember 2020.)

National Institute on Drug Abuse. (2020a) Costs of substance abuse. Retrieved from https://www.drugabuse.gov/drug-topics/trends-statistics/costs-substance-abuse. (Accessed 7 September 2020.)

National Institute on Drug Abuse. (2020b). Misuse of prescription drugs research report. Retrieved from https://www.drugabuse.gov/download/37630/misuse-prescription-drugs-research-report.pdf?v=add4ee202a1d1f88 f8e1fdd2bb83a5ef. (Accessed 7 September 2020.)

Peplau, H. (1951). *Interpersonal relations in nursing.* New York: G.P. Putman's Sons.

Platt, F.W., & Gordon, G.H. (2004). *Field guide to the difficult patient interview* (2nd ed.). Philadelphia: Lippincott, Williams, & Wilkins.

Raj, Y.P. (2020). Somatic symptom & related disorders. In M.D. Feldman & J.F. Christensen (Eds) *Behavioral medicine* (p. 322). New York: McGraw Hill.

Recovery Research Institute. (n.d.) Addictionary. Retrieved from https://www. recoveryanswers.org/addiction-ary/. (Accessed 7 September 2020.)

Reinhart, R.J. (2020). Nurses continue to rate highest in honesty, ethics. Retrieved from https://news.gallup.com/poll/274673/nurses-continue-rate-highest-honesty-ethics.aspx. (Accessed 7 September 2020.)

Rollnick, S., Miller, W.R., & Butler, C. (2008). *Motivational interviewing in health care. Helping patients change behavior.* New York: Gilford Press.

Schub, T.B., & Smith, N.R.M.C. (2017). Emotional intelligence in professional nursing practice. CINAHL Nursing Guide. Retrieved from https://www. ebscohost.com/nursing/products/cinahl-databases/cinahl-complete. (Accessed 7 September 2020.)

Shea, S.C. (2019). *The medication interest model: How to talk with patients about their medications.* Philadelphia: Wolters Kluwer.

Sherman, M.D., Miller, L.W., Keuler, M., et al. (2017). Managing behavioral health issues in primary care: 6 five-minute tools. *Family Practice Management,* 24(2), 30–35.

Smith, P., Schmidt, S., Allensworth-Davies, D., & Saitz, R. (2010). A single-question screening test for drug use in primary care. *Archives of Internal Medicine,* 170(13), 1155–1160.

Stokowski, L.A., McBride, M., & Berry, E. (2019). Medscape nurse career satisfaction report 2018. Retrieved from https://www.medscape.com/slideshow/2018-nurse-career-satisfaction-report-6011115. (Accessed 7 September 2020.)

Stuart, G.W. (2009). *Principles and practice of psychiatric nursing.* St. Louis, MO: Mosby Elsevier.

Substance Abuse and Mental Health Services Administration. (n.d.). *SBIRT: Screening, brief intervention, and referral to treatment.* Rockville, MD: SAMHSA.

Substance Use-Disorder Prevention that Promotes Opioid Recovery and Treatment for Patients and Communities Act. (2018). Public Law 115-271, October 24, 2018. Retrieved from https://www.congress.gov/115/plaws/publ271/plaw-115publ271.pdf. (Accessed 7 September 2020.)

Sue, K. (2020). The clinician's role: Reducing harm among people who use drugs. *The Carlat Addiction Treatment Report,* 8(1), 1, 4, 6.

Sulzer, S.H. (2015). Does "difficult patient" status contribute to de facto demedicalization? The case of borderline personality disorder. *Social Science & Medicine,* 142, 82–89.

Vago, D.R., & Silbersweig, D.A. (2012). Self-awareness, self-regulation, and self-transcendence (S-ART): a framework for understanding the neurobiological mechanisms of mindfulness. *Frontiers in Human Neuroscience,* 6, 1–30.

Vallis, M., Piccinini-Vallis, H., Sharma, A.M., & Freedhoff, Y. (2013). Clinical review: modified 5 As: minimal intervention for obesity counseling in primary care. *Canadian Family Physician Medecin de Famille Canadien,* 59(1), 27–31.

Wehbe-Alamah, H., & Wolgamott, S. (2014). Uncovering the mask of borderline personality disorder: knowledge to empower primary care providers. *Journal of the American Association of Nurse Practitioners,* 26(6), 292–300.

Wilson, N., Kariisa, M., Seth, P., Smith, H. IV, & Davis, N.L. (2020). Drug and opioid-involved overdose deaths – United States, 2017–2018. *Morbidity and Mortality Weekly Report (MMWR),* 69, 290–297.

Wlodarczyk, J., Lawn, S., Powell, K., et al. (2018). Exploring general practitioners' views and experiences of providing care to people with borderline personality disorder in primary care: A qualitative study in Australia. *International Journal of Environmental Research and Public Health,* 15(12), 2763.

Zulman, D.M., Haverfield, M.C., Shaw, J.G., et al. (2020). Practices to foster physician presence and connection with patients in the clinical encounter. *JAMA,* 323(1), 70–81.

Practical Considerations when Prescribing Controlled Substances

7

Pamela Stitzlein Davies

> This chapter discusses practical approaches to build expertise in prescribing controlled substances. A uniform approach to assessment of a patient prior to prescribing is advocated. Clinical guidelines and practice standards are reviewed. Terms related to drug use or misuse are defined and their application around complex issues discussed. Identification of patients who are at increased risk for substance use disorder is described, with "exit strategies" to utilize if the harm of therapy outweighs the benefit. The chapter presents the critical knowledge and skills necessary for the advanced practice registered nurse to become a comfortable and competent controlled substances prescriber.

Controlled substances (CSs) are powerful agents with specific prescribing restrictions. When used appropriately they can have a positive impact on quality of life, pain, function, mood, and sleep. When prescribed inappropriately they may be physically, emotionally, or socially harmful. It is important for the advanced practice registered nurse (APRN) to be a knowledgeable, competent, and astute prescriber of these drugs. Some APRNs choose not to prescribe CSs out of fear of adverse consequences and challenging situations. The analogy to fire is useful – fire can be both good and bad; when used appropriately, fire can warm a house, but if used recklessly it may burn it down.

Key issues for the APRN prescriber of CSs involve not only knowledge but also specific skills. This chapter addresses the practical considerations to be a competent prescriber. Critical areas are patient assessment, consistent follow-up and monitoring, use of guidelines and consensus statements, consideration of both the benefit and potential harms, and recognition of "red flags" related to CS use, with strategies for management.

DEFINITIONS RELATED TO CONTROLLED SUBSTANCES

In the United States, *legend* drugs are those requiring a prescription from an appropriately licensed provider. *Controlled substances* are medications regulated by the federal Controlled Substances Act of 1970 – drugs that have been

The Advanced Practice Registered Nurse as a Prescriber, Second Edition. Edited by Louise Kaplan and Marie Annette Brown.
© 2021 John Wiley & Sons Ltd. Published 2021 by John Wiley & Sons Ltd.

determined to be of higher risk for abuse and diversion. Schedule I drugs, such as heroin, are illegal. Schedule II drugs, such as morphine, are considered to have the highest risk of abuse, and no refills are allowed; a new prescription must be issued each time. Schedule III, IV, and V drugs represent progressively lower risk of abuse or diversion, and refills are allowed (Box 7.1). To prescribe CSs, health professionals must register with the Drug Enforcement Administration (DEA).

Box 7.1 Controlled substance schedules

Schedule I drugs are illegal under United States federal law and have "no currently accepted medical use and a high potential for abuse."

- Examples: heroin, ecstasy, marijuana*

Schedule II drugs have "a high potential for abuse, with use potentially leading to severe psychological or physical dependence" and are "considered dangerous."

- Requires original (hard copy) paper prescription or Electronic Prescription for Controlled Substance (EPCS)
- Prescription may not be telephoned or faxed to the pharmacy (except in limited circumstances)
- No refills allowed
- Additional restrictions in quantity may be added by individual states or third party payers
- Examples: morphine, oxycodone, fentanyl, hydrocodone compounds, cocaine, methylphenidate, methamphetamine

Schedule III, IV, and V drugs have moderate to low potential for dependence and abuse.

- Prescriptions may be telephoned or faxed to the pharmacy
- Schedule III and IV drugs may be refilled up to five times within six months of the date of issue of the original prescription
- Schedule V drugs may be refilled as authorized by the prescriber
- Examples of different classes:

  o Schedule III: Codeine (<90 mg) combined with another agent (such as acetaminophen with codeine), testosterone, ketamine
  o Schedule IV: tramadol (Ultram), alprazolam (Xanax), diazepam (Valium), carisoprodol (Soma), butorphanol (Stadol), zolpidem (Ambien)
  o Schedule V: Codeine cough syrup, Lomotil, pregabalin (Lyrica)

*Note: In the United States, marijuana remains illegal under federal law. However, some individual states have legalized medical or recreational marijuana use. See Chapter 9 on marijuana.

Sources: DEA- 2010, n.d.-a, n.d.-b.

It is critically important for APRNs to utilize the appropriate terms related to CS use and misuse in order to communicate professionally with colleagues and to document accurately. Box 7.2 lists common definitions. Improper use of these terms creates confusion. For example, clinicians may misapply the

---

Box 7.2 Definitions related to controlled substances

Abuse: Any use of an illegal drug or the intentional self-administration of a medication for a non-medical purpose such as altering one's state of consciousness, for example, getting high.

Addiction: is a treatable, chronic medical disease involving complex interactions among brain circuits, genetics, the environment, and an individual's life experiences. People with addiction use substances or engage in behaviors that become compulsive and often continue despite harmful consequences. Prevention efforts and treatment approaches for addiction are generally as successful as those for other chronic diseases.

Diversion: the intentional removal of a medication from legal dispensing and distribution channels.

Misuse: Use of a medication (for a medical purpose) other than as directed or indicated, whether willful or unintentional, and whether harm results or not.

Physical dependence: Engenders abstinence syndrome when the drug is abruptly stopped.

Tolerance: A state of adaptation in which exposure to the drug results in diminution of its effect over time.

Sources: American Society of Addiction Medicine, 2019; Webster, 2017.

---

term "addiction" when "tolerance" or "physical dependence" is intended. For clarity, it is optimal to utilize the term "psychological dependence" rather than "addiction." This also assures that patients are educated about the benefits and risks of CSs. A "teachable moment" can occur when patients comment: "I don't want to take that drug because I'll become addicted." When we help patients understand the differences between physiological and psychological dependence they may be more open to discussion of the medication (St. Marie, 2019). A key component of current language is use of the term "opioid" rather than "narcotic," as the former may have less negative associations.

THE OPIOID EPIDEMIC
The United States is facing an unprecedented crisis of opioid-related overdose deaths. These casualties have quadrupled in the last 15 years and nearly one-third of the deaths are related to valid prescriptions (Centers for Disease Control and Prevention [CDC], 2020a; Frieden & Houry, 2016). A historical perspective is helpful to understand how the current situation developed.

The historical cycle of treating pain in the United States: a swinging pendulum
Use of opioids for management of pain has varied widely in terms of acceptance, practice, guidelines, and laws over the last century to produce a "swinging

pendulum" effect (Mandell, 2016). In 1954, the Eisenhower administration created a cabinet committee "to stamp out narcotic addiction." The Nixon administration's "War on Drugs" led to passage of the *Comprehensive Drug Abuse Prevention and Control Act of 1970* and creation of the DEA in 1973. Healthcare providers were warned against the dangers of "creating addicts" if opioids were given (Mandell, 2016). Eventually, alarming reports began to circulate with tales of grossly inadequate management of patients with cancer dying in severe pain while opioids were withheld because of fear of creating addiction.

Clinicians witnessed how patients suffered in this overly restrictive environment. Attitudes of healthcare professionals, policy makers, and the public moved towards more liberal perspectives in the 1990s. Pain experts spoke out against the fear, avoidance, and stigmatization of opioids for management of acute and cancer pain (Wilkerson et al., 2016). Prominent experts promoted acceptance, even encouragement, of a more open-minded strategy towards prescribing opioids for chronic non-cancer pain (Veterans Health Administration/ Department of Defense [VA/DoD], 2017). Pharmaceutical companies played a significant role by vigorously promoting opioids and withheld information about the risk of psychological dependence in pain management (Quinones, 2015).

In 2001 the US Congress enacted the *Decade of Pain Control and Research*. The goals of this legislation were to raise awareness of inadequate pain control, improve treatments, and increase funding for research on pain. The decade saw many advances in the neuroscience of pain, new technologies for diagnosis and treatment of pain, and emergence of the role of complementary medicine in pain management. Campaigns by the American Pain Society in 1995 and the VA in 1999 endorsed the concept of "pain as the 5th vital sign" to promote frequent assessment of pain in both inpatient and outpatient healthcare settings in an endeavor to improve pain control (Levy et al., 2018; Wilkerson et al., 2016).

The prescribing of opioids was liberalized significantly, especially in the United States with only 5% of the world population while dispensing 75% of the prescription opioids (Shiffman, 2018). A decade of devastating opioid overdose deaths ensued. By the middle of the 2010s, the pendulum swung back towards a more restrictive opioid prescribing environment in the United States (Quinones, 2015).

The opioid overdose epidemic

The United States is in the midst of an unprecedented epidemic of drug overdose deaths. Between 1999 and 2017 a staggering 700,000 persons died from a drug overdose; 450,000 of these deaths involved an opioid (including both prescription and illicit opioids) (CDC, 2019). In 2017–2018 alone, more than 70,000 drug overdose deaths occurred and nearly 70% involved an opioid. This reflects a slight reduction from prior years, possibly due to recent legislative modifications and reductions in opioid prescribing (Figure 7.1). The overdose deaths have occurred in three "waves." The first wave started in the 1990s primarily related to prescribed opioids and was attributed to more liberal attitudes towards prescribing opioids for chronic pain. In 2010, the second wave of opioid-related overdose deaths emerged, primarily from heroin use – which is much lower cost. This was followed by the third wave in 2013 with the emergence of illicitly manufactured fentanyl, a powerful synthetic opioid analgesic (CDC, 2020a).

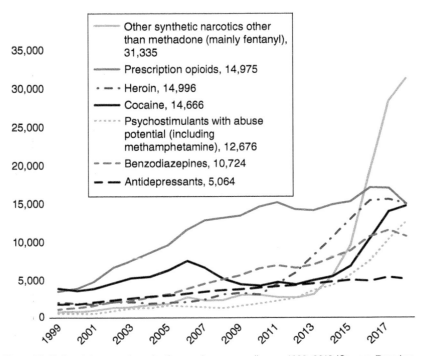

Figure 7.1 National drug overdose deaths, number among all ages, 1999–2018 (*Source:* Based on National Institute on Drug Abuse, 2020).

These reports reflect intentional and unintentional overdoses, and the involved drugs were legally prescribed, illegally obtained, or a combination. The majority of opioid-related deaths were not single-agent deaths but involved multi-substance exposure. An essential point for prescribers is to understand that the risk of overdose increases exponentially when opioids are combined with central nervous system depressants including benzodiazepines and alcohol (Figure 7.2) (Dowell et al., 2016; National Institute on Drug Abuse, 2020).

BEST PRACTICES WHEN PRESCRIBING CONTROLLED SUBSTANCES

Because it is impossible to determine with accuracy which clients will develop problems from CSs, a standardized approach to prescribing is needed. When patients are screened carefully prior to their initial prescription and vigilantly monitored during therapy, risk is decreased. The astute prescriber remains vigilant for problematic behaviors and should always keep an "exit strategy" in mind – that is, a plan to discontinue the medication if it appears the harm outweighs the benefits.

A universal approach

Just as healthcare providers use universal precautions to prevent transmission of infectious diseases, a helpful approach when prescribing CSs is to utilize *Universal Precautions in Pain Medicine* (Gourlay et al., 2005). This offers a

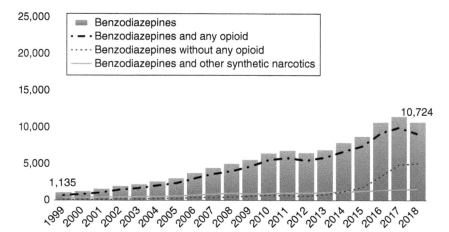

Figure 7.2 National drug overdose deaths involving benzodiazepines, by opioid involvement, number among all ages, 1999–2018 (*Source:* From Centers for Disease Control and Prevention, National Center for Health Statistics. Multiple Cause of Death 1999–2018 on CDC WONDER Online Database, released January, 2020. Public Domain).

standardized approach to management of opioids and other CSs. Patients are assessed for mood and substance use disorders, a treatment agreement is used, and they are followed carefully over time. Providers skillfully evaluate and document patient responses (Box 7.3).

Box 7.3 Universal precautions in pain medicine

- Make a diagnosis with an appropriate differential diagnosis
  - Identify conditions amenable to non-opioid therapies; periodically review the diagnosis and comorbid conditions
- Psychological assessment including risk of addictive disorders
  - Assess for depression, anxiety, post-traumatic stress disorder, and other mood disorders; include evaluation for substance use disorder or opioid use disorder; determine the risk for misuse and abuse; periodically update this review
- Informed consent
  - Discuss anticipated benefits and specific risks associated with the opioid or other CS (see Box 7.9)
- Treatment agreement
  - Review expectations and obligations of both the prescriber and the patient; this may include specific instructions for management of common or serious side effects, such as constipation or respiratory depression (see Box 7.9)
- Monitoring
  - Ongoing assessment of pain level and function
  - Standard monitoring strategies also include review of the state PDMP, periodic UDT, regular provider visits, and compliance with adjunct therapies such as physical therapy, counseling, and use of adjunctive medications or treatments

---

- Therapeutic trial
  - Emphasize that initiation of opioids or other CSs are a therapeutic trial and that continuation will depend on meeting clinical goals and appropriate utilization of non-pharmacological and other pharmacological therapies
- Documentation – Use of a standardized charting strategy such as the "5-As" to address important elements of follow-up assessments
  - Analgesia (pain intensity, or for non-opioid CSs substitute the primary symptom such as "anxiety," "insomnia," or "hyperactivity")
  - Activity (whether functional goals are being met)
  - Adverse effects (constipation, nausea, sedation)
  - Aberrant behavior (any evidence of misuse or abuse, lost prescriptions, review of the state Prescription Drug Monitoring Program, urine drug screen results)
  - Affect (mood, sleep)

Each CS prescription should be recorded in the medical record along with a notation that the state Prescription Drug Monitoring Program was reviewed.

Source: Modified from Gourlay et al., (2005).

Risk stratification and referral

An element of universal precautions is to stratify patients into one of three levels of care based on the risk of misuse or abuse of the CS to be prescribed. Placement of a patient in a particular level reflects the provider's expectation of what type of ongoing monitoring will be most appropriate. This process is meant to keep the patient and prescriber safe and maintain clinical practice within standards of care.

Risk stratification when prescribing CSs is detailed below (Bree Collaborative, 2018; VA/DoD, 2017):

Level 1: Primary Care

- Appropriate for lowest risk patients with no personal or family history of substance use disorder and no major or untreated behavioral health problems. Expert consultation may be sought if needed.

Level 2: Primary Care with Specialist Support

- Patients with a past personal or family history of substance use disorder; current behavioral health problems such as untreated or poorly controlled depression, anxiety, post-traumatic stress disorder, schizophrenia, or personality disorder. These patients are at moderate to moderate–high risk of inappropriate drug-related behaviors. The primary care provider is encouraged to consult and co-manage care with input from a specialist.

Level 3: Specialty Management

- Patients with active substance use disorder or severe untreated behavioral health problems who are at high risk of aberrant behaviors related to use of CSs. These complex patients should be referred for the aspects of care related to the problem for which CSs are prescribed to an interdisciplinary pain management center or other appropriate specialty such as psychiatry, addiction, or sleep medicine. APRNs should not attempt to manage these CS prescriptions unaided.

Specialist referral may be hindered by an insufficient number of experts; in some cases it may take months to obtain an appointment for a patient evaluation (Stanos et al., 2016). This creates a challenge for the primary care provider in need of expert assistance to manage the complexities of a Level 2 or 3 patient. Clinicians are encouraged to identify unique community resources such as consultation with a tertiary referral center via telehealth meetings that are designed to support general practitioners (Washington State Agency Medical Directors Group [WSAMDG], 2015a). The APRN can be more successful with high-risk patients if they can recognize and openly address the common strategies often employed by persons with active substance use disorder in an attempt to obtain CS prescriptions. APRNs can learn simple responses and effective strategies to respond to angry or tearful demands. Clinicians must stand firm and focus on care and comfort – yet defer CS prescriptions to a knowledgeable specialist.

Consistent utilization of a universal approach for patient care helps in the detection of potential for CS misuse. Although patients may express concerns about such assessments, explanations that all individuals are screened equally can reassure the patient and support the practitioner to proceed in a routine, systematic manner. These discussions will be most effective when approached in an open and respectful manner (Bree Collaborative, 2020).

CLINICAL GUIDELINES AND CONSENSUS STATEMENTS

Familiarity with major government and professional association guidelines and consensus statements related to utilization of CSs will help the provider remain informed of current practice standards and policies. Participation in national and local professional organizations offers opportunities for up-to-date knowledge about key policies or state laws and rules related to CS prescribing.

Opioid guidelines

In recent years, the efficacy of chronic opioid therapy (COT) for chronic non-cancer pain has been questioned due to lack of evidence to support this therapy, especially in the face of an epidemic of overdose deaths (Dowell, et al., 2016; WSAMDG, 2015a). A core feature of recent guidelines is to increase function rather than eliminate pain, as most studies do not show significant improvement in pain from COT (Busse et al., 2018; Chou, 2019). The provider's goal is to maximize safety for prevention of opioid overdose, limit opioid dose escalation, avoid combinations of opioids with benzodiazepines and other sedatives, and prescribe naloxone for emergency treatment of overdose in higher risk situations (Bree Collaborative, 2020; VA/DoD, 2017). See Box 7.4 for factors that increase adverse outcomes of opioid therapy.

CDC opioid prescribing guideline

All clinicians should be familiar with the Centers for Disease Control and Prevention (CDC) *Guideline for Prescribing Opioids for Chronic Pain – United States – 2016* (Box 7.5) (Dowell et al., 2016). When APRNs follow these recommendations, they can prescribe opioids in a judicious manner and remain alert

---

Box 7.4 Risk factors for adverse outcomes or overdose from opioid therapy

- Addiction disorders
  - o Diagnosis of substance use disorder or opioid use disorder
  - o Evidence of diversion of CSs
- Prescribing factors
  - o Higher opioid dose; any dose of opioid may potentially result in overdose but the risk increases over 50 morphine milligram equivalent (MME) per day and particularly over 100 MME per day
  - o Co-administration of benzodiazepines
  - o Longer duration of opioid therapy
  - o Methadone prescribed by novice practitioners
  - o Opioid naïve patient
- Medical conditions
  - o History of drug overdose
  - o Obstructive sleep apnea or other sleep-disordered breathing, severe respiratory instability, chronic pulmonary disease
  - o Renal disease
  - o Heart failure
  - o Cerebrovascular disease
  - o Drug or alcohol use disorders
- Mental disorders
  - o Suicidality
  - o Major depression
  - o Anxiety disorder
  - o Post-traumatic stress disorder
  - o Bipolar disorder
  - o Schizophrenia
  - o Borderline or antisocial personality disorder
- Patient factors
  - o Age younger than 30
  - o Recent release from prison
- Recent release from abstinence-based addiction treatment.

Sources: Dowell et al., 2016; VA/DoD, 2017; WSAMDG, 2015a; Webster, 2017.

---

to patient behaviors that warrant closer monitoring or consultation. Those who do not prescribe opioids should be familiar with the CDC guidelines to help monitor patients who have been prescribed opioids by other prescribers.

Key points of the CDC recommendations for COT for chronic pain include the importance of non-pharmacological and non-opioid pharmacological therapy for pain with realistic expectations for improvement in pain and function. Caution is important when prescribing COT *at any dose*. Safety considerations include careful reassessment at doses of 50 MME per day and avoidance of doses over 90 MME per day without thorough justification. The risk of accidental overdose from COT is significantly increased with concurrent benzodiazepine use and should be avoided if possible (Dowell et al., 2016).

Box 7.5 Centers for Disease Control and Prevention (CDC) recommendations for prescribing opioids for chronic pain outside of active cancer, palliative, and end-of-life care. (Note: Bold highlights by the author.)

Determining When to Initiate or Continue Opioids for Chronic Pain

1. **Non-pharmacologic therapy and non-opioid pharmacologic therapy are preferred for chronic pain.** Clinicians should consider opioid therapy only if expected benefits for both pain and function are anticipated to outweigh risks to the patient. **If opioids are used, they should be combined with non-pharmacologic therapy and non-opioid pharmacologic therapy,** as appropriate.

2. Before starting opioid therapy for chronic pain, clinicians should **establish treatment goals** with all patients, including **realistic goals for pain and function,** and should **consider how therapy will be discontinued if benefits do not outweigh risks.** Clinicians should continue opioid therapy only if there is **clinically meaningful improvement in pain and function** that outweighs risks to patient safety.

3. Before starting and periodically during opioid therapy, clinicians should discuss with patients the known **risks and realistic benefits of opioid therapy** and patient and provider responsibilities for managing therapy.

Opioid Selection, Dosage, Duration, Follow-Up, and Discontinuation

4. **When starting opioid therapy for chronic pain,** clinicians should **prescribe immediate-release opioids instead of extended-**release/long-acting (ER/LA) opioids.

5. When opioids are started, clinicians should **prescribe the lowest effective dosage.** Clinicians should use caution when prescribing opioids at any dosage, should carefully reassess evidence of individual benefits and risks when increasing dosage to ≥50 morphine milligram equivalents (MME) per day, and should avoid increasing dosage to ≥90 MME per day or carefully justify a decision to titrate dosage to ≥90 MME per day.

6. Long-term opioid use often begins with treatment of acute pain. **When opioids are used for acute pain,** clinicians should prescribe the lowest effective dose of immediate-release opioids and should prescribe no greater quantity than needed for the expected duration of pain severe enough to require opioids. **Three days or less will often be sufficient; more than seven days will rarely be needed.**

7. Clinicians should **evaluate benefits and harms with patients within one to four weeks of starting opioid therapy** for chronic pain or of dose escalation. Clinicians should evaluate benefits and harms of continued therapy with patients **every three months** or more frequently. **If benefits do not outweigh harms of continued opioid therapy, clinicians should optimize other therapies and work with patients to taper opioids to lower dosages or to taper and discontinue opioids.**

Assessing Risk and Addressing Harms of Opioid Use

8. Before starting and periodically during continuation of opioid therapy, clinicians should evaluate risk factors for opioid-related harms. Clinicians should incorporate strategies to mitigate risk, such as offering naloxone, into the management plan. History of SUD, higher opioid dosages (≥50 MME per day) or concurrent benzodiazepine use reflect high risk.

9. Clinicians should review the patient's history of controlled substance prescriptions using state prescription drug monitoring program (PDMP) data to determine whether the patient is receiving opioid dosages or dangerous combinations that put him or her at high risk for overdose. **Clinicians should review PDMP data when starting opioid therapy for chronic pain and periodically during opioid therapy for chronic pain, ranging from every prescription to every three months.**
10. When prescribing opioids for chronic pain, clinicians should use urine drug testing before starting opioid therapy and consider UDT at least annually to assess for prescribed medications as well as other controlled prescription drugs and illicit drugs.
11. Clinicians should avoid prescribing opioid pain medication and benzodiazepines concurrently whenever possible.
12. Clinicians should offer or arrange evidence-based treatment (usually medication assisted treatment with buprenorphine or methadone in combination with behavioral therapies) for patients with **opioid-use disorder.**

Source: Dowell et al., 2016.

The CDC website contains a useful online educational series, with 13 modules containing information on the CDC opioid recommendations, treating chronic pain without opioids, communicating with patients, motivational interviewing techniques, and other topics (CDC, 2020b). Free continuing education credits are available until April 2022.

Veterans Health Administration and Department of Defense opioid therapy clinical practice guidelines

The VA/DoD have pioneered numerous clinical practice guidelines on a variety of topics such as low back pain, chronic insomnia, and substance use disorder which the primary care provider in any setting will find useful in daily practice (VA/DoD, 2020). The VA/DoD *Clinical Practice Guideline for Opioid Therapy for Chronic Pain* contains helpful algorithms and recommendations for pain management with a focus on biopsychosocial assessment and management (VA/DoD, 2017). Key points include recommendations *against* the initiation of COT for chronic pain, especially in people younger than 30 years old, and *against* the concurrent use of benzodiazepines with opioids, and recommendation for suicide screening prior to initiation of COT.

Washington State opioid guideline

The Washington state *Interagency Guideline on Prescribing Opioids for Pain* website has several very useful tools:

- An interactive web-based Opioid Dose Calculator to determine MMEs
- Assessment and screening tools
- A list of "red flags" indicating further work-up is needed
- A detailed interpretation algorithm for use in urine drug testing (UDT)
- Educational videos (WSAMDG, 2015b).

Also from Washington State, the Bree Collaborative *Opioid Prescribing: Long-Term Opioid Therapy Report and Recommendations* imparts a practical approach for prescribers of COT. The emphasis is on important practice approaches such as the development of a respectful relationship, assessment of patient knowledge and discussion of realistic expectations of pain care, and validation of patient concerns, all with a consistent message. After assessment, patients should be stratified into three treatment pathways: maintain current opioid dose and monitor regularly, taper opioid, or transition to medications for opioid use disorder (Bree Collaborative, 2020).

CLINICAL GUIDANCE FOR BENZODIAZEPINES AND OTHER CONTROLLED SUBSTANCES

There are few formal clinical practice guidelines on prescribing benzodiazepines, benzodiazepine receptor agonists, stimulants, or other CSs in adults. Nonetheless, these drugs are frequently overprescribed and are not carefully monitored in most settings (Grossbard et al., 2014).

Benzodiazepines and benzodiazepine receptor agonists

Benzodiazepines significantly increase the risk of overdose and death when combined with opioids; this combination should be avoided whenever possible, especially in chronic use (Dowell et al., 2016). The overdose risk is significantly increased if alcohol or other sedative-hypnotic agents are added.

In older adults, use of benzodiazepines and benzodiazepine receptor agonists (BZRA or "Z-drugs" such as zolpidem) is of particular concern due to the associated increased risk of falls, fracture, delirium, motor vehicle accidents and increased risk of death (Canadian Coalition for Seniors' Mental Health, 2019; Pottie et al., 2018). Reduced renal clearance associated with aging contributes to these risks; acute illness, dehydration, or drug interactions can significantly exacerbate the problem. Both classes of drugs have long been listed on the American Geriatric Society's *Beer's Criteria for Potentially Inappropriate Medication Use in Older Adults* (American Geriatrics Society Beers Criteria Update Expert Panel, 2019). Nonetheless, use of these drugs in the aged remains widespread, and is a significant source of morbidity and mortality (Markota et al., 2016).

Stimulants

Stimulants, such as methylphenidate and dextroamphetamine, are used for treatment of attention deficit hyperactivity disorder (ADHD) in children and adults. They are reported as a highly effective and safe treatment of ADHD and are recommended in current clinical practice guidelines in conjunction with behavioral interventions (Wilens & Kaminski, 2020; Wolraich et al., 2019).

As Schedule II drugs, stimulants have been determined to hold a high potential for abuse. Although the majority of patients use them appropriately, non-medical use of stimulants has increased. Those at highest risk of abuse are white males 18–25 years old. Signs of abuse may include substance use disorder, academic decline, and psychopathology. Atomoxetine is an alternative effective non-stimulant legend agent with a lower abuse potential. Although many high-school and college students request stimulants to improve study skills, non-medical use of stimulants is associated with lower grades and is also correlated with abuse of alcohol (64%), marijuana (44%), cocaine (10%), and other agents (Wolraich et al., 2019).

Clinicians are encouraged to utilize best practices to prescribe stimulants for ADHD to reduce misuse and diversion (Wilens & Kaminski, 2020; Wolraich et al., 2019).

- Be aware of patients at risk for non-medical use and diversion of stimulants and consider alternative pharmacological therapies.
- Discuss safe storage of medicines and prevention of diversion, and explain the ethical and legal consequences of diverting drugs; ideally, this can be accomplished with a medication agreement.
- Prescribe only sufficient quantities for use so that none is left to stockpile; consider prescribing less than a 30-day supply.

ASSESSMENT OF PATIENTS PRIOR TO INITIATING A CONTROLLED SUBSTANCE

The importance of thorough patient assessment as the essential foundation for diagnosis and a plan of care cannot be overemphasized. Other factors, especially the risk of CS misuse, are mandatory to evaluate when prescribing CSs.

Patient history

Selection of a CS prescription to manage pain or other issues such as anxiety, insomnia, or hyperactivity requires a comprehensive history, with assessment of the primary symptom such as pain location, intensity, character, exacerbating and relieving factors, radiation, and temporal factors. Additionally, the patient should be queried about the impact of pain or other symptoms on mood, sleep, work, relationships, sexuality, recreation, and overall functioning. Inquire about personal or family history of smoking, alcohol, substance use, and psychiatric problems such as untreated depression or anxiety, post-traumatic stress disorder, bipolar disorder, schizophrenia, and personality disorder. Presence of these conditions stratifies the patient to a higher risk category for CS misuse (Box 7.4) (Webster, 2017). Additional evaluation should be done to detect comorbid conditions that may affect prescribing a CS. For example, the presence of untreated sleep apnea could affect the safe use of an opioid or benzodiazepine.

Because alcohol is such a ubiquitous part of US culture, patients and providers can easily dismiss its use and overuse in a review of risk or lifestyle factors. Careful assessment of alcohol use is needed since it is the most common substance misused in the United States and increases the risk of overdose when mixed with sedating CSs (Addiction Campuses, 2018; Dowell et al., 2016).

Even if a chronic condition has required a CS for years, it is essential to regularly assess for "red flags" that may indicate other health problems that warrant further evaluation. Examples include:

- New neurological deficits
- Personal history of malignancy (especially lung, breast, and prostate cancers that are more likely to have osseous metastasis)

- Sudden change in the nature of the pain complaint
- Constitutional symptoms such as unexplained weight loss of 20 pounds or more
- Fevers, chills, night sweats, or excessive fatigue (Verhagen et al., 2016).

In most cases when a CS is under consideration, the patient interview should be augmented by screening tools and self-administered questionnaires specific to the condition. See Box 7.6 for suggested instruments, many of which are available online.

Box 7.6 Screening and monitoring tools for controlled substance prescribing

- Screening for Risk of Opioid Misuse
  - Opioid Risk Tool for Opioid Use Disorder (ORT-OUD)
    - Nine-item tool with yes or no responses
    - May be self-administered, but best data are obtained from interview along with correlation by review of the medical record
    - Assessing personal and family history of alcohol, drug, or prescription drug abuse; age between 16 and 45; and mental health conditions
    - Each positive item gets one point, a score of 3 or higher indicates increased risk of opioid misuse
    - Does not assess for the higher risk items of smoking and post-traumatic stress disorder (PTSD)
  - Screening and Opioid Assessment for Persons with Pain, Revised (SOAPP-R)
    - 24-item tool with four response options
    - Self-administered; takes about eight minutes
    - Assesses personal, family, and friends' history of alcohol or drug abuse, mood swings, sense of boredom, tension at home, running out of medicines early, craving
    - Score of 18 or higher indicates increased risk of opioid misuse
- Ongoing Compliance on Opioid Therapy
  - Opioid Compliance Checklist (OCC)
    - Eight-item checklist with yes or no responses
    - Self-administered
    - Asks if opioids taken other than prescribed, run out of pain medication early or lost pills, used illicit substances
    - A score of 1 or more predicts the likelihood of future opioid misuse
- Alcohol and Other Substance Use
  - CAGE Adapted to Include Drugs (CAGE-AID)
    - Four-item tool with yes or no responses
    - Interview or self-administered
    - Originally developed to screen for alcoholism, adapted to include drug use
    - CAGE is an acronym for: Cut down, Annoyed, Guilty, Eye-opener based on the following questions:
      - "Have you ever felt you ought to cut down on your drinking or drug use?"
      - "Have people annoyed you by criticizing your drinking or drug use?"
      - "Have you ever felt bad or guilty about your drinking or drug use?"
      - "Have you ever had a drink or used drugs first thing in the morning ['eye-opener'] to steady your nerves or to get rid of a hangover?"
    - One or more affirmative responses is a positive screen for alcohol or drug use problems

---

- o Alcohol Use Disorders Identification Test – Concise (AUDIT-C)
  - Three-item questionnaire, each item scored 0–4
  - Self-administered
  - Asks about the frequency, quantity, and pattern of alcohol intake
  - A score of 4 or more for men or 3 or more for women is a positive screen
- Mental Health Screening
  - o Patient Health Questionnaire (PHQ)
    - Depression screen utilized in many settings
    - Two-question (PHQ-2) or nine-question (PHQ-9) versions with four response options
    - Two-item screen asks about "Little interest or pleasure in doing things" and "Feeling down, depressed, or hopeless" in the last two weeks
    - A score of 3 or more on PHQ-2 is positive; on PHQ-9, a score of 5, 10, 15, or 20 are cutoffs for mild, moderate, moderate–severe, or severe depression
  - o Generalized Anxiety Disorder (GAD)
    - Anxiety screen utilized in many settings
    - Two-question (GAD-2) or seven-question (GAD-7) versions with four response options
    - Two-item screen asks about "Feeling nervous, anxious, or on edge" and "Not being able to stop or control worrying" in the last two weeks
    - A score of 3 or more on GAD-2 is positive; on GAD-7 a score of 5, 10, or 15 are cutoffs for mild, moderate, or severe anxiety
  - o Primary Care Post-Traumatic Stress Disorder (PC-PTSD)
    - Five questions with yes or no responses
    - Asks about nightmares, easily startled, feelings of detachment and self-blame
    - A score of 3 or more is a positive screen
- Pain Assessment
  - o Pain intensity, Enjoyment of life and General activity (PEG)
    - Three-item tool, with responses on a patient's 0–10 scale
    - Self-administered
    - Used for tracking response to therapy and pain interference over time; a lower score is better
  - o Fibromyalgia Screening Tool
    - Includes Widespread Pain Index (WPI) and Pain Catastrophizing Scale (PCS)
    - 40-item tool
    - Self-administered
    - WPI includes a body diagram with 19 regions to indicate areas of pain or tenderness in the last seven days
    - A Symptom Severity scale assessing fatigue, cognitive and sleep problems over the last seven days, as well as abdominal pain, depression, or headache in the last six months
    - PCS lists 13 statements reflecting fear of pain, with five response options
- Sleep Apnea Screening
  - o STOP-BANG tool (Snore-Tired-Obstruction-Pressure, BMI-Age-Neck-Gender)
    - Reviews risk factors for sleep apnea which may increase the incidence of adverse respiratory effects for patients taking opioids or sedative-hypnotics.

Sources: Brown et al., 2017; Cheatle et al., 2019; Jamison et al., 2016; National HIV Curriculum, 2020; Oregon Pain Guidance, 2020; St. Marie, 2019; WSAMDG, 2015a.

It is also important to obtain and review records from current or past providers to assess previous diagnostic work-ups and past trials of non-pharmacological and pharmacological therapies for the condition. Because past behavior is predictive of future actions, specific attention should be given to patient adherence with the plan of care for previous CS prescriptions, particularly any history of aberrant behaviors such as unexpected findings in urine drug screens or on the PDMP. Clinicians are encouraged to defer writing CS prescriptions until a full review of past records is completed, as it can provide important insights that impact decision making (Gourlay et al., 2010). The review of past history should be documented in the medical record.

Physical examination

The physical examination should fully address the specific complaint, such as a complete neurological exam for complaint of headache, or thorough musculoskeletal exam, especially spine palpation, range of motion, gait, lower extremity strength, sensation, and reflexes for low back pain.

Physical signs of drug abuse should be assessed particularly when prescribing a CS. These include:

- Track marks – scars from needle use in the antecubital space or other venous access sites on arms, legs, between toes, or neck
- Skin popping – scars from subcutaneous injection of drugs, usually on arms
- Nasal septal perforation from cocaine use
- Mentation changes such as nodding off during the visit from medication oversedation
- Pupil size – unexpectedly small or large pupil size.

Diagnostic testing

Laboratory and diagnostic tests should be pursued as needed to establish the diagnosis and rule out other conditions. For example, a complaint of increased anxiety may include assessment of thyroid function, metabolic panel, complete blood count, and electrocardiogram. A significant change in the quality or frequency of headaches may prompt brain imaging to ensure that no serious condition has developed. Renal function should be ascertained whenever prescribing a drug to older adults. Intravenous drug use is the most common route to acquire hepatitis C, with 50% of persons who inject drugs exposed to it (Shiffman, 2018). Hepatitis C may serve as a proxy to identify substance use disorder and some guidelines recommend testing for hepatitis C prior to prescribing CSs as an approach to identify high-risk behaviors (American Association for the Study of Liver Diseases and the Infectious Diseases Society of America, 2019; VA/DoD, 2017).

State Prescription Drug Monitoring Programs

In the United States, PDMPs are state-administered electronic databases that track CS prescriptions. Authorized providers in all states and many territories of the United States can access a PDMP. Some states require, and all guidelines urge, review of the database prior to a new prescription (CDC, 2020c). In some cases it is possible to view prescriptions across state lines, which is helpful for coordination of care.

The PDMP is a safety tool that can help reduce overdose risk and promote responsible prescribing (DEA, 2019). One study found that at least half of fatal overdoses could be identified retrospectively based on multiple prescribers, multiple pharmacies, and daily doses of 100 MME or more (Baumblatt et al., 2014). A review of all CS prescriptions issued to a patient allows providers to easily discover these risk factors as well as multiple drugs in the same class and dangerous drug combinations, such as opioids combined with benzodiazepines (CDC, 2020). Such findings represent a "red flag" that requires additional exploration to assess for inappropriate use of COT and other CSs.

Challenges with PDMP may exist due to cumbersome access to the system or delays in posting data. However, significant improvements have been made in recent years, particularly integration of the PDMP with the electronic medical record (EMR) in many healthcare systems, along with more current data (CDC, 2020). However, problems with access to timely data still exist for some federal medical facilities (e.g. Indian Health Services, US Department of Veterans Affairs) and prisons. A major gap in the PDMP is the lack of information from opioid treatment programs such as methadone maintenance and buprenorphine clinics (American Society of Addiction Medicine, 2018). Major safety concerns exist when patients do not reveal their participation in medication assisted therapy, which may be withheld due to understandable concerns such as fear of provider stigma.

Urine drug testing

Despite weak evidence, most clinical guidelines recommend UDT and it is now standard protocol for COT in many primary and specialty care settings (Kale, 2019; Mahajan, 2017). Although appropriate to monitor UDT when prescribing non-opioid CSs, it is not commonly done in practice. Testing may identify a previously undiagnosed substance use disorder, which can be as high as 30% in some patient cohorts (VA/DoD, 2017). Prior to the initiation of an opioid, UDT should be performed to identify patients with current substance use (e.g. findings of cocaine or metabolites of heroin) or those at higher risk for opioid overdose (e.g. unanticipated findings of benzodiazepines or alcohol) (Dowell et al., 2016). This informs the clinician about patients who would benefit from more frequent monitoring or those who are not appropriate for CSs. In one large cohort, patients most likely to show aberrant UDT results are males, smokers, age younger than 45, and those with history of substance use disorder (Turner et al., 2014). Although some may express concern about UDT, assurance that UDT is a universal requirement for all patients receiving CSs may reduce distress. Inclusion of information about UDT in the patient care agreement can provide education and normalize the testing.

For ongoing surveillance, UDT results supplement patient self-report and serve to verify adherence to the treatment plan. Although not fool-proof, UDTs identify the presence or absence of expected (prescribed) drugs and unexpected drugs (illicit drugs or those not prescribed). This can facilitate honest discussions with the patient and aid clinicians with their decisions about ongoing care (Turner et al., 2014).

Frequency of UDT varies according to patient risk factors, policies in the care setting, and state policy. The CDC recommends UDT a minimum of annually for those on COT (Dowell et al., 2016). The Washington State opioid guidelines recommend UDT frequency based on risk stratification for opioid and CS misuse (WSAMDG, 2015a):

- Low risk: every 6–12 months
- Moderate risk: every 3–6 months
- High risk: every 1–3 months.

There are two types of UDTs available: an immunoassay and comprehensive (confirmatory) assay (see Box 7.7) (Gourlay et al., 2010). Costs for UDT vary by lab, locale and type of tests performed. UDT is a covered expense with Medicare and most insurance plans in the US, although some will not cover the cost of both types of UDT when obtained at the same visit (Mahajan, 2017). The window of detection for most opioids is 1-3 days after ingestion. To aid in test interpretation, query the patient about when the last dose was taken (Kale, 2019). UDTs are ideally performed randomly, and some clinics require that patients report to the lab for a UDT within 24 hours of a request. However, in practical terms, this may be a significant challenge for patients to accommodate due to distance to the health center, access to transportation, work schedule, or childcare or elder care responsibilities.

Box 7.7 Urine drug testing assays

Test	Immunoassay	Comprehensive/confirmatory
Overview	Basic screening test detects only naturally occurring opiates (morphine), cannabinoids, cocaine, and amphetamines. Specialized immunoassays (available in some settings) can detect additional drugs including synthetic or semisynthetic opioids (oxycodone, hydrocodone, fentanyl, methadone), benzodiazepines, or barbiturates.	Comprehensive test which detects synthetic and semisynthetic opioids in addition to naturally occurring opiates; benzodiazepines, barbiturates, and other drugs of abuse. Uses gas or liquid chromatography and mass spectrometry (GC/MS or LC/MS). Provides confirmatory testing for a basic screening UDT.
Advantages	Rapid results (minutes to hours). May be available as "point of service" (in clinic). Lower cost.	More sensitive. Provides a "true positive" or "true negative." Often includes a formal interpretation by a laboratory toxicologist which is helpful for clinical decision making when unexpected results are obtained.
Limitations	Potential for false-positive or false-negative results and cross-reaction with other agents. Provider must be familiar with the drugs that can actually be detected by the test used in the clinic.	Higher cost. Results and interpretation may take several days.

Sources: Gourlay et al., 2010; Kale, 2019; Mahajan, 2017.

UDT can be confusing to interpret. For example, codeine is metabolized to morphine and hydrocodone in small quantities and may be found in the confirmatory UDT results (Box 7.8). The metabolite 6-monoacetylmorphine is a precursor to morphine and would lead the provider to suspect heroin use rather than morphine, as heroin metabolizes in minutes but the heroin metabolite may be present in urine for 12–24 hours after injection (VA/DoD, 2017). Therefore an established consultative relationship with the laboratory toxicologist will aid in proper interpretation of test results. Expert input should be obtained prior to making treatment decisions based on UDT results, especially if the plan is to taper and discontinue the CS. The Washington State opioid guidelines have extensive information on UDT in the appendix, to aid in the interpretation of test results, particularly decision algorithms, and UDT clinical vignettes (WSAMDG, 2015a).

Box 7.8 Urine drug screen interpretation: selected opioid metabolites

Drug	Urinary metabolites
Codeine	Codeine, possibly morphine and hydrocodone
Methadone	Methadone
Morphine	Morphine, possibly hydromorphone
Hydrocodone	Hydrocodone, possibly hydromorphone
Hydromorphone	Hydromorphone
Oxycodone	Oxycodone, possibly oxymorphone
Heroin	6-monoacetylmorphine is pathognomonic for heroin use
	Morphine, possibly codeine
	(Note: heroin is seldom detected as the half-life is only three to five minutes)

Sources: VA/DoD, 2017; WSAMDG, 2015a.

Consultation

As with any other aspect of practice, it is essential that providers understand the limitations of their knowledge and seek input from specialists when needed. Novice providers in particular are encouraged to seek consultation as an indicator of careful, quality care in light of the complexity of chronic opioids, benzodiazepines, or other CSs. Informal consultation with a trusted colleague can provide perspective and direction. Formal consultation with a pain medicine clinic, mental health provider, or addictionologist is essential for complex cases.

The clinician is advised to collaborate with the consultant in the development of a pharmacological treatment plan that is feasible within the primary care environment. Many pain specialists will make recommendations for therapy but will not assume primary responsibility for prescribing opioids on a chronic basis. Similarly, some psychiatrists will provide consultation on pharmacological management of psychiatric problems but will not prescribe CSs on an ongoing basis. Clear communication with the consultant is essential to clarify who is the primary prescriber.

Diagnosis

When initiating a prescription for a CS, the medical diagnosis should be as specific as possible based on findings in the history, physical examination, and diagnostic tests. For example, spinal stenosis or myofascial tenderness is preferred over the generic term "back pain."

INITIATING CONTROLLED SUBSTANCE PRESCRIPTIONS

After careful evaluation the provider may determine that the benefits of prescribing a CS outweigh the risks and thus move forward with informed consent and development of a plan to initiate therapy. In most cases CS therapy should *not* be started at the first visit with a patient. A few weeks are usually needed to obtain and review past medical records, especially if the patient has received a CS in the past. An important piece of information about whether to prescribe a CS in the future may be obtained from a UDT performed at the initial visit. The patient should be seen in person at a subsequent visit to initiate the first CS prescription which will allow time to review and sign the treatment agreement and answer questions.

Managing patient expectations

Skills to manage patient expectations can be readily learned and used as part of the informed consent process. Persons on COT for chronic non-cancer pain typically report no more than a 20–30% decrease in pain intensity (Bree Collaborative, 2020). In conjunction with a multimodal plan of care, improvements in function, sleep, mood, and social interactions are the primary goals of COT rather than a reduction in pain. Patients must understand that CSs for symptom management are *never* the sole therapy. Non-pharmacological management strategies (such as mindfulness meditation or regular exercise) must be continued for optimal results, along with other pharmacotherapy as appropriate for the condition. While written information about CSs is useful, a significant amount of time is needed to educate patients about the risks, benefits, and realistic expectations for CS therapy.

Treatment agreements

Prior to prescribing CSs on a long-term basis, the expectations and responsibilities of the provider and patient should be clearly communicated, with an emphasis on the consequences if patient responsibilities are unmet. Although there is no evidence that utilization of a controlled substance treatment agreement (CSTA) will decrease CS misuse or abuse (McAuliffe Staehler & Palombi, 2020), the agreements can nonetheless be most helpful to facilitate communication about key aspects of care (Rager & Schwartz, 2017). CSTAs are most commonly employed for patients on COT but may be adapted for use with other agents such as benzodiazepines, sedative-hypnotics, or stimulants (Ait-Daoud et al., 2018).

There are an array of CSTA examples which vary in length from half a page to several pages. Ideally, the agreement will address these key aspects (Tobin et al., 2016):

- Informed consent (risks and benefits of therapy)
- Promotion of safe use and reduction of aberrant behaviors
- Expectations for patient behavior (such as obtaining CS prescriptions from one provider, using a single pharmacy, keeping physical therapy and other referral appointments, abstaining from alcohol use, and submitting to random urine drug testing)
- Patient education.

CSTAs enhance the process of shared decision making (Tobin et al., 2016). They also function as an important educational tool for management of possible drug side effects such as constipation or sedation, driving safety concerns, instructions for drug safekeeping in the home, potential drug interactions, and naloxone use (Dunn et al., 2017). Additionally, inclusion of standard clinic policies will prevent patients from being taken unaware. Two particular policies require special emphasis: three business days for renewals and no replacement of lost or stolen prescriptions. A standardized approach should be utilized for all patients to provide consistency and not to single out any particular patient or patient group (Rager & Schwartz, 2017). Although not essential, a patient signature ensures that the document was actually viewed by the patient. A written copy should be provided to the patient for future reference. Box 7.9 describes items commonly included in opioid or CS agreements, with weblinks to samples.

Initial dosing

In most cases, the prescriber should initiate therapy with the lowest dose available and titrate slowly over a period of days to weeks to the target dose (Dowell et al., 2016). For those who are known to be particularly sensitive to drug side effects and for older adults, consider starting with one-half of the lowest tablet strength for one to two weeks. Many providers communicate frequently with patients during the titration phase. This process can be facilitated by scheduled telephone visits with the clinic nurse or requesting the patient to send messages via the electronic health record on a weekly basis for a few weeks.

Below is an example of a slow titration schedule to initiate methylphenidate for multiple sclerosis-related fatigue in a patient known to have problems with insomnia and anxiety.

- Therapy is initiated with one-half of a 5-mg tablet (2.5 mg) taken once in the morning for three to seven days.
- If this dose is tolerated but is subtherapeutic, the patient is instructed to increase the dose to 5 mg each morning, or alternatively, take one-half of a 5-mg tablet (2.5 mg) twice a day at breakfast and lunch for one to two weeks and report results by phone or e-message.
- If this dose is tolerated but symptoms are not significantly improved, the patient is instructed to increase to 5 mg in the morning and 2.5 mg at lunch for one to two weeks and report results again.
- Since the initial target dose is 5–20 mg per day, depending on how the patient responds to therapy, further escalation of dose may be appropriate, using a similar stepwise approach.

Box 7.9 Examples of content that may be included in opioid or controlled substance treatment agreements

Informed Consent
- Goals of therapy
  - For chronic opioid therapy, the focus is on improved function rather than reducing pain
- Risks and benefits of treatment
- Alternatives to proposed treatment with a CS

Expectations and Responsibilities of the Patient
- Use only one prescriber or prescriber group for the CS therapy
- Keep the provider advised of all current medications, including other CSs
- Do not obtain opioids or other CSs from other sources unless specifically discussed and approved by the provider
  - Notify the clinic of any temporary CS prescriptions (such as emergency department or dental visit)
- Utilize a single pharmacy
- Use the CS only as prescribed, do not change the dose or frequency of medication without approval
- Keep regularly scheduled follow-up appointments
  - Specify the typical follow-up intervals for the clinic (e.g. every three months)
- Agree to discuss concerns in a calm and respectful manner, will not yell, be verbally abusive, or use threatening language to any staff member
- Keep appointments with specialists as referred, such as physical therapy, social work, psychiatry
- Actively work on progress toward functional goals such as physical therapy exercises, aerobic activity, mindfulness practice
- Honesty regarding medical history, including substance use history
- Agree to sign requests for outside records and understand that CSs will not be prescribed from this office until records are reviewed
- Agree to inform provider of changes in health status or possibility of pregnancy
- Agree to avoid all illicit drugs, non-prescribed drugs, or recreational drugs
  - Specify clinic policy regarding use of cannabis
- Agree to submit a sample for UDT when requested and within the time frame requested
- Understand consequences of failing to uphold the expectations of the agreement
- Be provided with a description of behaviors that will result in discontinuation of drug

Clinic Policies
- Allow three business days for prescription renewal requests
- No renewals on evenings, weekends, or holidays
- "No early refill" policy
- No replacement of lost or stolen prescriptions
- PDMP database will be reviewed prior to issuance of prescriptions, and any irregularities may result in delay of prescription renewal
- Unexpected findings in the urine drug screen will be sent for confirmatory testing, which may have financial impact for the patient
  - Findings of cocaine, methamphetamine, or heroin metabolites in the urine drug confirmatory test will result in immediate discontinuation of the CS
  - Findings of other unexpected agents (non-prescribed CS, absence of prescribed drug) in the urine test will require an interim in-clinic visit with the provider before the next renewal
- Patients must provide a valid phone number or a contact person and must respond within one business day if requested

Patient Education
- When and where to call for questions or problems
- Expected side effects and management of side effects
  - Opioid therapy should include information on constipation, sedation, cognitive changes, dry mouth, endocrine system changes (amenorrhea, infertility, hypotestosteronism)
- Driving safety and work safety related to potential cognitive changes from sedating drugs
- Avoid dangerous drug combinations such as alcohol or sedating drugs
  - Increased risk of overdose when opioids are combined with benzodiazepine and/ or alcohol
- Concerning signs and symptoms of problems that may be caused by the prescribed CS
  - Excessive sedation, cognitive problems, manic behaviors
- Instruction on naloxone purpose and importance of filling the prescription
  - Provide written instructions for family/caregiver on how and when to administer naloxone for suspected opioid overdose

Safekeeping of Drugs
- Do not give, share, or sell drugs to others
- Keep drugs locked in a safe place to avoid them being taken by family, friends, visitors
- Treat the pills like cash, do not leave them out on the kitchen or bathroom counter
- Dispose of CSs properly, including unused tablets or capsules or used patches or oralets

Sample treatment agreement forms can be viewed at:

Oregon Pain Guidance, Patient Treatment Agreements: https://www.oregonpainguidance.org/app/content/uploads/2016/05/patient-treatment-agreements.pdf.

National Institute on Drug Abuse, Sample Patient Agreement Forms: https://www.drugabuse.gov/sites/default/files/files/samplepatientagreementforms.pdf.

Child, Adolescent and Adult Psychiatry – Center for ADHD, Controlled Substances Treatment Agreement: http://www.centerforadhd.com/controlled-substances-agreement.pdf. (Accessed 7 September 2020.)

Sources: Dowell et al., 2016; Liu, 2020; Philpot et al., 2017; Tobin et al., 2016.

Usually, there is no need for a rapid titration of a CS for chronic conditions. Because there may be wide variation in patient response to therapy, a cautious approach is required to prescribe a new CS. In the example above, one patient may respond to a dose of 2.5 mg once daily, and another patient may be optimized at 20 mg twice a day. Until the clinician gains experience, it is best to start a new CS prescription with a low dose and titrate slowly, especially in older patients and patients who are more sensitive to drugs. The APRN is also advised to consult with a pharmacist for patients with impaired renal function.

Therapeutic trial

Initiation of therapy with a CS should be a deliberately planned and thoughtful intervention. Initially it is considered a *therapeutic trial* for a designated period of time, for example, two weeks to three months (VA/DoD, 2017). Together the patient and provider need to establish the criteria for a successful trial of a CS drug and determine what constitutes "clinically meaningful" improvement in symptoms. For example, improved functional level and decreased interruptions of sleep due to pain may be realistic goals for a patient with chronic low back pain who begins opioid therapy. The 2016 CDC opioid guideline indicates that patients who do not experience a "clinically meaningful" response to opioids early in therapy, such as at one month, are unlikely to experience improvement with longer use (Dowell et al., 2016). Pain relief should not be the primary goal of COT, as "clinically meaningful" pain reduction is unlikely to occur in the long term (Chou, 2019). Patient expectations must be refocused towards improved function and other "clinically meaningful" goals.

If a therapeutic trial does not meet the goals during the target period, the drug should be tapered and discontinued (Dowell et al., 2016). In some cases, it may be appropriate to extend the trial for an additional one to two months. If so, a very clear end date must be set to assure that CSs do not inadvertently become a chronic but ultimately ineffective and potentially dangerous therapy. Alternative CS therapies may be tried if troublesome side effects are encountered. Other non-CS pharmacological agents, such as anticonvulsants for neuropathic pain, and non-pharmacological therapies, such as mindfulness practice, should be continued throughout the CS therapeutic trial. The VA/DoD Clinical Practice Guideline (2017) has a helpful algorithm in Module B to initiate a therapeutic trial of opioids.

Approach to new patients who are currently taking controlled substances

Addressing the needs of a patient who is new to the provider and already taking a CS on a regular basis can be challenging. There are three situations in which this occurs: new patients to the clinic who have never been seen before and are transferring their care; the "inherited patient" who is established in the clinic but is transferring care from another provider; and providing temporary coverage for another provider in the same clinic who is on vacation or extended leave. Suggested approaches to these situations are listed below.

New patients

Many providers and clinics follow the recommended approach and establish a policy that they will not prescribe CSs at the initial visit for patients new to the clinic. Ideally, this information is communicated verbally when the initial patient appointment is scheduled and also stated on written clinic intake forms. Deferment to a future visit allows time to obtain and review outside records for any history of aberrant drug taking behaviors. If additional information is needed, the clinician is encouraged to speak directly with the previous provider. Obtain a signed release of information for past medical records as well as permission to speak with past providers. The PDMP should also be reviewed to determine what CSs have actually been dispensed.

Patients may seek care with the expectation of a CS prescription at the first visit, and, indeed, may need it to prevent withdrawal. However, the provider has no obligation to prescribe a CS until a thorough assessment has determined that it is safe to do so. This does not represent patient abandonment, as the relationship is not yet established and the clinician has not made the determination of whether the CS prescription is appropriate. Patients who are at risk of withdrawal may be referred back to their previous prescriber for a one to two months' prescription until a review has been completed.

Clinicians are advised to stand firm in their decision not to prescribe at the initial visit. It is much easier never to prescribe an inappropriate therapy than it is to stop one after it has been started – even one that was supposed to be temporary. It would serve the APRN well to be proactive and work with clinic leadership to create a policy to address these situations and provide consistent team communication throughout the intake process.

The "inherited patient"

The "inherited patient" refers to an established patient at the clinic with a transfer of care from another provider who has left the position (Gourlay & Heit, 2009). Similar to the decision of whether to continue a controversial therapy, such as chronic use of a proton pump inhibitor for non-specific gastric complaints, the clinician must determine whether a CS regimen is appropriate for this particular patient. Although the provider may not concur with the use of a controlled drug, there is nonetheless a responsibility to continue with the current plan of care in the short term (weeks to months) because the patient has established care at the clinic.

As the new prescriber of the CS, the APRN now takes on the responsibility for the risks and benefits of therapy. Therefore it is prudent to:

* Review all previous records
* Thoroughly evaluate the problem that precipitated the need for the CS
* Review the diagnostic work-up performed
* Consider additional evaluation or consultation
* Review past PDMP and UDT reports
  o Assess for evidence of aberrant patient behaviors
* Update the CSTA with new provider and patient signatures
* Provide education and dialogue with the patient about any concerns.

The new clinician may determine that the current therapy is appropriate and should continue unchanged, or instead may assess that it is in the patient's best interest to taper to a lower dose or discontinue the agent altogether. If the latter is recommended, the clinician should thoroughly explain the concerns, answer questions in detail, and give the patient time to adjust to the new recommendations. Unless there are urgent safety concerns, the revised CS prescribing plan should be gradually implemented, over weeks to months (Bree Collaborative, 2020; US Department of Health and Human Services [HHS], 2019a).

Coverage for colleagues

Lastly, it is common practice to write prescriptions for the patients of colleagues while they are temporarily on vacation or leave. First assess the PDMP for CS prescriptions in the past few months. Also review the last UDT results and ensure that a CSTA is in place. Challenges arise when irregularities exist (such as cocaine noted in a previous UDT that was never addressed by the primary prescriber) or the dose or quantities exceed current guidelines. In most cases, the clinician should continue the previous plan of care, but any identified concerns should be carefully documented. Consideration can be given to writing only a partial prescription, such as a 14-day instead of the usual 28-day supply, until the usual prescriber returns. Below is a documentation example for a coverage situation:

> Vacation coverage for Dr Jane Doe, APRN, for renewal of oxycodone CR. Chart briefly reviewed. Last UDT (confirmatory) dated 5/20/2020 noted to have cocaine and unprescribed morphine, but appears the issue has not yet been addressed as Dr Doe is out of the office. PDMP congruent, CSTA on file dated 8/2019. Pt will be out of medication in 2 days.

> Plan: Will continue with Dr Doe's current plan of care, but due to findings in recent UDT will provide only a 14-day supply. Pt must come in for follow-up appointment with Dr Doe within 2 weeks to discuss UDT results. Attempted to reach patient by phone to discuss findings, no answer, left message requesting he call back. Informed RN of situation, request she try to reach patient and schedule follow-up.

Options for future therapy

When meeting a new or "inherited" patient, there are three approaches the clinician may take to assume the provider role for CS prescriptions:

1. maintain and monitor,
2. taper or discontinue, or
3. transition to treatment for opioid or substance use disorder (Bree Collaborative, 2020).

After the patient assessment and records review, careful consideration should be given to the appropriateness of continuing the therapy at the current or a reduced dose. If the CS appears to be contributing to improved quality of life and function without significant adverse effects or risks, the option of maintaining the therapy with ongoing monitoring can be considered. This may take a few months of observation to determine. For patients who may benefit from ongoing CS therapy but are receiving excessive doses, the clinician should discuss safety concerns and recommend a taper to a lower dose. Negotiating details of the taper with the patient can help them feel empowered in the process and improve success (HHS, 2019a). A targeted date for reaching the lower dose should be clearly established. Additional information on tapering CS medication is detailed below.

There is often considerable variability across providers in their approaches to CSs. It is essential for APRNs to understand that they are not obligated to prescribe a CS to any patient for which it appears to be unsafe or unsound practice. Guidance from the medical director and clinic manager should be sought when uncomfortable situations occur. Development of a clinic-wide policy for handling such situations can be most helpful for all providers, especially novices.

Patients who are resistant to evaluation, necessary diagnostic testing (including UDT), and review of past records, despite explanatory discussions, are not appropriate for therapy with CSs (Gourlay et al., 2010). For additional guidance see Chapter 6, "Managing Difficult and Complex Patient Interactions."

Naloxone for management of opioid overdose

The CDC recommends that providers offer patients naloxone to mitigate the risk of fatal opioid overdose. The risks of overdose are increased with higher opioid doses ($\geq$50 morphine equivalent daily dose), concurrent benzodiazepine use, history of substance use disorder, or prior overdose (Dowell et al., 2016). Medical conditions that may increase the risk of opioid overdose include sleep apnea and some psychiatric conditions (American Medical Association Opioid Task Force, 2017). It is essential that education about recognition of opioid overdose be provided to the patient as well as the family members, caregivers, or cohabitants who are most likely to administer this life-saving therapy. They should be taught that signs of opioid overdose may include shallow and slow respirations with snoring or gurgling sounds, inability to arouse, blue or gray lips or fingernails, and very small pupils (American Society of Anesthesiologists, n.d.).

The rescuer should be instructed to administer naloxone and call emergency services for assistance. Even if the patient revives after naloxone administration, it has a short half-life and additional doses will likely be needed. Naloxone is available as a nasal spray or auto-injector. Every state has access to naloxone at pharmacies through statewide protocols/pharmacist prescriptions, statewide standing orders, or laws that allow naloxone to be dispensed without a prescription (National Alliance of State Pharmacy Associations, 2019). Educational brochures can be found online.

DEA "X" license

Medication assisted therapy (MAT) with buprenorphine or methadone for treatment of opioid use disorder (OUD) requires a DEA "X" license. This specialized license is in addition to a valid DEA authorization to prescribe Schedule II–V drugs. In many states, APRNs may apply for a "buprenorphine waiver" to treat OUD after they complete 24 hours of mandatory education and meet certain requirements (Substance Abuse and Mental Health Services Administration, 2020). Methadone for OUD may only be administered or dispensed as part of a comprehensive opioid treatment center (e.g. "methadone maintenance" therapy) (Substance Abuse and Mental Health Services Administration, 2015).

Despite these restrictions, methadone and buprenorphine may both be prescribed for analgesia by any provider with a DEA license for Schedule II drugs. The clinician must carefully assess the patient to assure that the goals of pharmacotherapy are for analgesia and that they are not inadvertently (and illegally) treating OUD. This is particularly important for methadone as MAT doses may not appear high when compared to morphine doses. Analgesic doses for methadone are generally in the range of 5–20 mg daily in divided doses, whereas MAT doses range from 60 to 120 mg once daily.

MONITORING OF PATIENTS RECEIVING CONTROLLED SUBSTANCE PRESCRIPTIONS

Patients who take a CS need to be monitored on a regular basis. A standardized approach to documentation will enhance the likelihood of a thorough assessment. Review of the diagnosis for which the CS is prescribed and repeat physical examination related to the condition should be performed annually and as needed to affirm the absence of other conditions, concerns, or "red flag" symptoms (Verhagen et al., 2016).

Frequency of visits

The CDC recommends surveillance of patients who receive COT every three months, or more frequently for those with higher risk conditions that may place them at higher risk of opioid overdose. Some clinics require monthly in-person visits to renew the CS prescription. This practice allows for frequent follow-up but may lead to scheduling concerns related to patient or provider illness or vacation. The policy works best in a group practice setting where clinician visits are shared.

Writing renewal prescriptions

Schedule II (CII) CSs cannot be refilled and require a new prescription for each dispensing, either the original ("hard copy") paper prescription or an electronic prescription for controlled substance (EPCS). Schedule III, IV, and V drugs may use EPCS or be faxed or "called in" to the pharmacy, and refills are allowed. See Box 7.1 for details (DEA n.d.-a, n.d.-b). Although DEA rules were modified in 2010 to allow electronic prescribing of CSs and it is approved in all US states (Villaseñor & Piscotty, 2016), the transition has been slow due to complexities and cost of integrating EMR software into the requirements of the EPCS. Many of these concerns have been recently addressed and electronic prescriptions of CSs have increased (O'Reilly, 2019).

In addition to federal (DEA) rules, many US states and third-party payers have implemented policies that impact opioid prescriptions for management of acute pain. For example, in Washington state opioid prescriptions are limited to a 7-day supply for acute pain, 7- to 14-day supply for acute postoperative phase of pain (depending on the professional commission), and 14-day supply for subacute phase of pain unless a clinical justification is provided. Additionally, Washington state Medicaid limits the quantity of tablets dispensed to opioid naïve patients to 18 tablets for those under age 21 and 42 tablets per 90 days for adults; after six weeks of therapy an attestation is required to continue. (Washington State Healthcare Authority, 2019). Each clinician must become familiar with individual state law and third-party payer rules in order to prescribe opioids and other CSs.

A variety of approaches exist when providers manage chronic CII prescriptions. Although the DEA does not limit the quantity of a CII drug dispensed, many states and third-party payers allow no more than a 30-day supply to be dispensed at a time. Procedures vary for renewal of CII prescriptions based on the individual prescriber preference and clinic or healthcare system policy (DEA, 2007, n.d.-c; Gabay, 2013; O'Reilly, 2019; Villaseñor & Piscotty, 2016). Examples include:

- Patients have monthly clinic visits and the CII prescription is renewed at each visit. If the patient does not keep the appointment, the CS is not typically renewed until the person has an appointment. This option is labor intensive but allows for close surveillance.
- Patients have asynchronous clinic visits every few months, but the clinic visit differs from the prescription renewal. Prescriptions are written one month at a time. If EPCS is not utilized, hard copy prescriptions must be mailed to the patient (which requires at least one full week of lead time to arrive before the supply runs out) or left at the front desk for pickup. This option requires patients to request prescriptions in a timely manner. It also allows for monthly review of the PDMP prior to issuance of each prescription.
- The DEA allows a prescriber to issue multiple CII prescriptions authorizing a patient to receive up to a 90-day supply. At the quarterly follow-up visit, the provider writes three one-month CII prescriptions. Each prescription must list the future fill date.
  - For example: prescription #1 is filled 8/4/2020, prescription #2 and #3 state "Do not fill until 9/1/2020" and "Do not fill until 9/29/2020" respectively.

Writing monthly CS prescriptions is time-consuming and requires organization. Many settings advocate issuance of CS prescriptions for a 28-day supply rather than 30-day. By using a four-week cycle, prescriptions are always renewed on the same day of the week (for example, every fifth Tuesday) and avoids situations where renewals are needed on weekends. This will help prevent last-minute urgent renewal requests and unpleasant or potentially dangerous symptoms related to acute withdrawal from opioids, benzodiazepines, or other CS. The PDMP is ideally, and in some states required to be, reviewed prior to each CS prescription renewal, but at a minimum every three months (Dowell et al., 2016).

Documentation
A strategy that promotes brief but inclusive clinical documentation is use of the "Five As of Pain Medicine" (Box 7.3) (Gourlay et al., 2005). This includes questions about analgesia, activity, adverse effects, aberrant behavior, and affect. The first item, analgesia, can be modified to assess the impact of other CSs. Additionally, each CS prescription should be recorded in the medical record along with notation when the state PDMP is reviewed.

STRATEGIES FOR TAPER AND DISCONTINUATION OF CONTROLLED SUBSTANCES

When prescribing CSs, the overall approach must include a predetermined plan to taper and discontinue the therapy if it becomes necessary. This is called an "exit strategy." Rationale for this action may include troublesome side effects (such as mania from stimulants), lack of attainment of clinically meaningful improvement goals (no functional improvement from opioids), or concerning behaviors (unexpected findings in the UDT). Using a CSTA that explains potential concerns and clearly delineates the consequences of aberrant behaviors will significantly assist with patient communication if discontinuation is necessary (Box 7.9).

Useful strategies to taper and discontinue CSs are to either schedule a clinic visit to address the concerns face-to-face with the patient and address questions or request a video or telephone conference. If the patient cannot be reached (usually associated with aberrant behaviors), a letter should be mailed and also sent via the EMR messaging system indicating that the CS must be discontinued, include a brief explanation, and encourage the patient to contact the office to discuss the situation further.

Clinicians are encouraged to continue to provide care for patients who must have the CS discontinued (Bree Collaborative, 2020). Most established patient–provider relationships can successfully continue when CSs are discontinued, although egregious behaviors or violations of trust, such as threatening the provider or prescription forgery, may sever the therapeutic relationship.

Standing firm in decision

Ideally, the determination to taper or discontinue a CS is a shared decision made with the patient and involved caregivers. However, in cases of patient safety in which the risks of therapy appear too high, the clinician can make a unilateral decision to stop the therapy (Bree Collaborative, 2020). For example, a patient on COT who is found to have both non-prescribed benzodiazepines and opioids in the UDT is at increased risk of opioid overdose. Despite careful discussion of the concerns, the patient may insist that the opioids be continued or even demand a dose increase. Because the provider may be intimidated by this situation, it is essential to clearly focus on established guidelines and stand firm. A helpful reminder is that safety is ultimately in the best interest of the patient. John Loeser, MD, professor emeritus at the University of Washington and former medical director of the Multidisciplinary Pain Clinic, offers his approach to tough clinical decisions about opioid dosing: "It's my ball and my ballpark and I make the rules!" (J. Loeser, personal communication, May 22, 2020). Despite his commitment to a strong patient–provider relationship, Dr Loeser argues that the final mantle of authority and responsibility related to CSs ultimately rests with the individual clinician who writes the prescription.

Self-care

Interactions surrounding discontinuation of CSs can occasionally create contentious debates, and strong emotions are experienced by all involved, including clinic staff. The clinician is encouraged to seek out a mentor for direction and support with difficult patient conversations. Discussions with one's confidential peer support systems can be very helpful. It is important to actively utilize self-care measures such as deep breathing, mindfulness meditation, aerobic exercise, and good sleep habits to optimize coping skills after a challenging day. Also see Chapter 6 for additional guidance.

Tapering controlled substances

A slow taper of the CS over a period of time is optimal, if safety considerations allow. Tapers may last a few days or weeks, or in the case of benzodiazepines or high-dose opioids can take months or more than a year to accomplish (Dowell et al., 2019).

The US Department of Health and Human Services (HHS) document *Guide for clinicians on the appropriate dosage reduction or discontinuation of long-term analgesics* provides practical strategies for opioid tapers. Taper schedules range from 5 to 20% dose reduction every month, with slower tapers better tolerated and more successful. It emphasizes that: "Tapers may be considered successful as long as the patient is making progress, however slowly, towards a goal of reaching a safer dose, or if the dose is reduced to the minimal dose needed" (HHS, 2019a, p. 3).

A taper can be stressful for patients. It is an opportunity to provide extra support and to initiate other therapies, both non-CS pharmacological and non-pharmacological. Patients who collaborate in the taper plan are more likely to be successful. Most patients will benefit from frequent check-ins with the provider or clinic nurse for reassurance and serving as a coach or cheerleader to affirm the patient's progress.

Misapplication of guidelines when tapering opioids

After release of the CDC "Guideline for Prescribing Opioids for Chronic Pain" (Dowell et al., 2016), unfortunate episodes of mismanagement due to misapplication of the guideline were reported. In a subsequent article addressing this issue, Dowell et al. recommend clinicians carefully consider each patient's unique situation when they seek guideline-concordant care (Dowell et al., 2019). Providers who dismiss patients from the practice based on the dose of their opioid therapy, or abandon prescribing opioids altogether, misunderstand the CDC opioid guidelines. The authors' take-home message is there are "no shortcuts to safer opioid prescribing" (Dowell et al., 2019, p. 1). It takes a considerable investment of professional growth and skill development to prescribe COT in a safe and effective manner.

HHS encouraged providers to "avoid misinterpreting cautionary dosage thresholds as mandates for dose reduction" (HHS, 2019a, p. 2). Additionally, clinicians are given the following warning:

"Risks of rapid tapering or sudden discontinuation of opioids in physically dependent patients include acute withdrawal symptoms, exacerbation of pain, serious psychological distress, and thoughts of suicide. Patients may seek other sources of opioids, potentially including illicit opioids, as a way to treat their pain or withdrawal symptoms. Unless there are indications of a life-threatening issue, such as warning signs of impending overdose, HHS does not recommend abrupt opioid dose reduction or discontinuation" (HHS, 2019a, p. 1).

Benzodiazepine taper

Canadian clinicians and researchers developed a very useful website, *deprescribing.org*, which provides clinician guidance and patient information brochures about deprescribing risky drugs in older adults (deprescribing.org, 2020). The site supports use of appropriate assessment strategies and provides the guidance to taper benzodiazepine and BZRA agents. Key recommendations for taper and discontinuation includes: 1) patient education on why deprescribing is necessary, with information on alternative non-pharmacological therapies (such as cognitive-behavioral therapy for management of insomnia or anxiety); and 2) a slow taper with frequent follow-up every one to two weeks (Pottie et al., 2018). Slow tapers over a period of months are more successful, with reduced relapse rates (Markota et al., 2016). Taper schedules typically involve a dose reduction of 25% every two weeks until the lowest dose is reached, then progressively adding drug-free days (Pottie et al., 2018). Abrupt discontinuation of chronic benzodiazepines should be avoided as it can induce seizures and may be potentially fatal. It is also frequently associated with rebound anxiety that can make future attempts to taper more difficult (Markota et al., 2016). Detailed examples of benzodiazepine taper schedules are provided in these references (Markota et al., 2016; Pottie et al., 2018).

Opioid use disorder and substance use disorder
OUD, affects several million Americans. It is defined as a "problematic pattern of opioid use leading to clinically significant impairment or distress" (Dowell et al., 2016, p. 32). All clinicians should be able to recognize behaviors that raise concerns for OUD and substance use disorder. Criteria for OUD are listed in Box 7.10. After discussion and education, patients who struggle with these concerns should be referred for specialized care (Schuckit, 2016).

A helpful mnemonic to recognize substance abuse is the "5 C's" (Gardner, 2008). This tool uses straightforward language that can be used to educate patients or family members when concerns arise about addiction. Persons with psychological dependence to a substance demonstrate:

- Impaired Control over use
- Compulsive use
- Continued use despite obvious harm to self and others
- Craving the substance
- Chronic condition.

In general, primary care clinicians should not prescribe CSs to patients with behaviors that raise concern for OUD or substance use disorder. In a situation where the patient is already receiving CSs, consultation with an experienced mentor or an addictionologist is advised.

CONCLUSION
As APRNs have gained broader prescriptive authority, they must also understand the complex issues and develop skills that enable them to safely prescribe CSs. This chapter has addressed methods to prescribe CSs in a way to avoid potential inappropriate use. While providers must approach CS prescribing with wisdom, vigilance and caution, it is absolutely essential to avoid fear and reluctance to prescribe CSs for the relief of human suffering. Guidelines provide directions for chronic non-cancer pain as well as other CSs. A standardized plan to prescribe CSs include a careful assessment, a universal approach to all patients, and use of a CSs treatment agreement. The astute clinician will provide a consistent approach to all patients who receive opioids or other CSs. This consistency may help avoid inappropriate prescribing, provide strategies to

---

Box 7.10 Criteria for diagnosis of opioid use disorder

In order to confirm a diagnosis of OUD, at least two of the following should be observed within a 12-month period:

- Opioids are often taken in larger amounts or over a longer period than was intended.
- There is a persistent desire or unsuccessful efforts to cut down or control opioid use.
- A great deal of time is spent in activities necessary to obtain the opioid, use the opioid, or recover from its effects.
- Craving or a strong desire or urge to use opioids.
- Recurrent opioid use resulting in a failure to fulfill major role obligations at work, school, or home.
- Continued opioid use despite having persistent or recurrent social or interpersonal problems caused or exacerbated by the effects of opioids.
- Important social, occupational, or recreational activities are given up or reduced because of opioid use.
- Recurrent opioid use in situations in which it is physically hazardous.
- Continued opioid use despite knowledge of having a persistent or recurrent physical or psychological problem that is likely to have been caused or exacerbated by the substance.
- Tolerance, as defined by either of the following: a need for markedly increased amounts of opioids to achieve intoxication or desired effect, or a markedly diminished effect with continued use of the same amount of an opioid. Note: This criterion is not met for individuals taking opioids solely under appropriate medical supervision.
- Withdrawal, as manifested by either of the following: the characteristic opioid withdrawal syndrome, or the same (or a closely related) substance is taken to relieve or avoid withdrawal symptoms. Note: This criterion is not met for individuals taking opioids solely under appropriate medical supervision.

Scoring
Mild: 2–3 items
Moderate: 4–5 items
Severe: 6 or more

Source: Based on Substance Abuse and Mental Health Services Administration, 2018.

---

deal with unexpected findings, and provide reassurance that the plan of care is within accepted standards. Although prescribing CSs can be complex and time-consuming, when appropriately prescribed, these drugs have the potential to improve the quality of life for persons with a variety of disorders.

REFERENCES

Addiction Campuses. (2018). Most commonly used addictive drugs in the U.S. Retrieved from https://www.addictioncampuses.com/blog/most-addictive-drugs/. (Accessed 7 September 2020.)

Ait-Daoud, N., Hamby, A.S., Sharma, S., & Blevins, D. (2018). A review of alprazolam use, misuse, and withdrawal. *Journal of Addiction Medicine*, 12(1), 4–10.

American Association for the Study of Liver Diseases and the Infectious Diseases Society of America. (2019). HCV guidance: Recommendations for testing, managing and treating hepatitis C. Retrieved from https://www. hcvguidelines.org. (Accessed 7 September 2020.)

American Geriatrics Society Beers Criteria® Update Expert Panel. (2019). American Geriatrics Society 2019 updated AGS Beers Criteria® for potentially inappropriate medication use in older adults. *Journal of the American Geriatrics Society*, 67(4), 674–694.

American Medical Association Opioid Task Force. (2017). Help save lives: Co-prescribe naloxone to patients at risk of overdose. Retrieved from https:// www.end-opioid-epidemic.org/wp-content/uploads/2017/08/ama-opioid-task-force-naloxone-one-pager-updated-august-2017-final-1.pdf . (Accessed 7 September 2020.)

American Society of Addiction Medicine. (2018). Public Policy Statement on Prescription Drug Monitoring Programs (PDMPs). Retrieved from https:// www.asam.org/quality-science/publications/magazine/public-policy-statements/2018/04/24/prescription-drug-monitoring-programs-(pdmps). (Accessed 7 September 2020.)

American Society of Addiction Medicine. (2019). Definition of addiction. Retrieved from https://www.asam.org/quality-science/definition-of-addiction. (Accessed 7 September 2020.)

American Society of Anesthesiologists. (n.d.). Opioid overdose resuscitation. Retrieved from https://www.asahq.org/whensecondscount/wp-content/uploads/2017/10/asa-opioid-overdose-resuscitation-guide-1.pdf. (Accessed 7 September 2020.)

Baumblatt, J.A.G., Wiedeman, C., Dunn, J.R., et al. (2014). High-risk use by patients prescribed opioids for pain and its role in overdose deaths. *JAMA Internal Medicine*, 174(5), 796–801.

Bree Collaborative. (2018). Collaborative care for chronic pain: report and recommendations. Retrieved from http://www.breecollaborative.org/topic-areas/previous-topics/chronic-pain/. (Accessed 7 September 2020.)

Bree Collaborative. (2020). Opioid prescribing: long-term opioid therapy report and recommendations. Retrieved from http://www.breecollaborative.org/topic-areas/previous-topics/opioid/. (Accessed 7 September 2020.)

Brown, R., Deyo, B., Riley, C., et al. (2017). Screening in Trauma for Opioid Misuse Prevention (STOMP): Study protocol for the development of an opioid risk screening tool for victims of injury. *Addiction Science & Clinical Practice*, 12(1), 28.

Busse, J.W., Wang, L., Kamaleldin, M., et al. (2018). Opioids for chronic noncancer pain: a systematic review and meta-analysis. *JAMA*, 320(23), 2448–2460.

Canadian Coalition for Seniors' Mental Health. (2019). Canadian guidelines on benzodiazepine receptor agonist use disorder among older adults. Retrieved from https://ccsmh.ca/wp-content/uploads/2020/01/benzodiazepine_receptor_agonist_use_disorder_eng_jan-24.pdf. (Accessed 7 September 2020.)

Centers for Disease Control and Prevention. (2019). Annual surveillance report of drug-related risks and outcomes. Retrieved from https://www.cdc.gov/drugoverdose/pdf/pubs/2019-cdc-drug-surveillance-report.pdf. (Accessed 7 September 2020.)

5445554544444444

Centers for Disease Control and Prevention. (2020a). Opioid overdose: understanding the epidemic. Retrieved from https://www.cdc.gov/drugoverdose/epidemic/index.html. (Accessed 7 September 2020.)

Centers for Disease Control and Prevention. (2020c). Prescription Drug Monitoring Programs (PDMPs). Retrieved from https://www.cdc.gov/drugoverdose/pdmp/states.html. (Accessed 7 September 2020.)

Centers for Disease Control and Prevention (2020b). Interactive training series for healthcare providers. Retrieved from https://www.cdc.gov/drugoverdose/training/online-training.html. (Accessed 7 September 2020.)

Cheatle, M.D., Compton, P.A., Dhingra, L., et al. (2019). Development of the revised opioid risk tool to predict opioid use disorder in patients with chronic nonmalignant pain. *The Journal of Pain*, 20(7), 842–851.

Chou, R. (2019). Opioids improve chronic noncancer pain, but difference may not be clinically meaningful in most patients. *Annals of Internal Medicine*, 170(8), JC41.

deprescribing.org. (2020). Creating evidence-based deprescribing guidelines. Retrieved from https://deprescribing.org/news/creating-evidence-based-deprescribing-guidelines/. (Accessed 7 September 2020.)

Dowell, D., Haegerich T.M., & Chou, R. (2016). CDC guideline for prescribing opioids for chronic pain – United States, 2016. *MMWR Recommendations and Reports*, 65(RR-1), 1–49.

Dowell, D., Haegerich, T., & Chou, R. (2019). No shortcuts to safer opioid prescribing. *New England Journal of Medicine*, 380(24), 2285–2287.

Drug Enforcement Administration. (2007). Issuance of multiple prescriptions for schedule II controlled substances. *Final rule. Federal Register*, 72(222), 64921–64930.

Drug Enforcement Administration. (2010). Part 1306 – Prescriptions. Controlled substances listed in Schedules III, IV, and V. §1306.22. Refilling of prescriptions. Retrieved from https://www.deadiversion.usdoj.gov/21cfr/cfr/1306/1306_22.htm. (Accessed 7 September 2020.)

Drug Enforcement Administration. (2019). Opioid overdose, information for providers. What healthcare providers need to know about PDMPs. Retrieved from https://www.cdc.gov/drugoverdose/pdmp/providers.html. (Accessed 7 September 2020.)

Drug Enforcement Administration- (n.d.-a). Drug scheduling-. Retrieved from https://www.dea.gov/drug-scheduling. (Accessed 7 September 2020.)

Drug Enforcement Administration (n.d.-b). Electronic prescriptions for controlled substances. Retrieved from https://www.deadiversion.usdoj.gov/resources.html. (Accessed 7 September 2020.)

Drug Enforcement Administration. (n.d.-c). Q&A. Retrieved from https://www.deadiversion.usdoj.gov/faq/prescriptions_faq.htm. (Accessed 7 September 2020.)

Dunn, K.E., Yepez-Laubach, C., Nuzzo, P.A., et al. (2017). Randomized controlled trial of a computerized opioid overdose education intervention. *Drug and Alcohol Dependence*, 173, S39–S47.

Frieden, T.R., & Houry, D. (2016). Reducing the risks of relief – the CDC opioid-prescribing guideline. *New England Journal of Medicine*, 374(16), 1501–1504.

Gabay, M. (2013). Federal Controlled Substances Act: controlled substances prescriptions. *Hospital Pharmacy*, 48(8), 644–645.

Gardner, E.L. (2008). Pain management and the so-called "risk" of addiction: A neurobiological perspective. In: H.S. Smith & S.D. Passik (Eds). Pain and chemical dependency (pp. 427–435). New York: Oxford University Press.

Gourlay, D.L. & Heit, H.A. (2009). Universal precautions revisited: managing the inherited pain patient. *Pain Medicine*, 10(Suppl 2), S115–S123.

Gourlay, D.L., Heit, H.A., & Almahrezi, A. (2005). Universal precautions in pain medicine: a rational approach to the treatment of chronic pain. *Pain Medicine*, 6(2), 107–112.

Gourlay, D.L., Heit, H.A., & Caplan, Y.H. (2010). Urine drug testing in clinical practice. The art and science of patient care, edition 4. Retrieved from https://www.healthcare.uiowa.edu/familymedicine/fpinfo/docs/drug%20screens%202015.pdf. (Accessed 7 September 2020.)

Grossbard, J.R., Malte, C.A., Saxon, A.J., & Hawkins, E.J. (2014). Clinical monitoring and high-risk conditions among patients with SUD newly prescribed opioids and benzodiazepines. *Drug and Alcohol Dependence*, 142, 24–32.

Jamison, R.N., Martel, M.O., Huang, C.C., et al. (2016). Efficacy of the opioid compliance checklist to monitor chronic pain patients receiving opioid therapy in primary care. *The Journal of Pain*, 17(4), 414–423.

Kale, N. (2019). Urine drug tests: ordering and interpreting results. *American Family Physician*, 99(1), 33–39.

Levy, N., Sturgess, J., & Mills, P. (2018). "Pain as the fifth vital sign" and dependence on the "numerical pain scale" is being abandoned in the US: why? *British Journal of Anaesthesia*, 120(3), 435–438.

Liu, Z. (2020). Prescription opioid misuse by family members: implications for nurse practitioners. *The Journal for Nurse Practitioners*, 16(5), 355–358.

Mahajan, G. (2017). Role of urine drug testing in the current opioid epidemic. *Anesthesia & Analgesia*, 125(6), 2094–2104.

Mandell, B.F. (2016). The fifth vital sign: A complex story of politics and patient care. *Cleveland Clinic Journal of Medicine*, 83(6), 400–401.

Markota, M., Rummans, T.A., Bostwick, J.M., & Lapid, M.I. (2016). Benzodiazepine use in older adults: dangers, management, and alternative therapies. *Mayo Clinic Proceedings*, 91(11), 1632–1639.

McAuliffe Staehler, T.M., & Palombi, L.C. (2020). Beneficial opioid management strategies: A review of the evidence for the use of opioid treatment agreements. *Substance Abuse*, 41(2), 208–215.

National Alliance of State Pharmacy Associations. (2019). Pharmacist prescribing: Naloxone. Retrieved from https://naspa.us/resource/naloxone-access-community-pharmacies/. (Accessed 7 September 2020.)

National HIV Curriculum. (2020). APRI calculator. Retrieved from https://www.hiv.uw.edu/page/clinical-calculators/apri. (Accessed 7 September 2020.)

National Institute on Drug Abuse. (2020). Overdose death rates. Retrieved from https://www.drugabuse.gov/related-topics/trends-statistics/overdose-death-rates. (.)

Oregon Pain Guidance. (2020). Assessment tools. Retrieved from www.oregonpainguidance.org/tools/. (Accessed 7 September 2020.)

O'Reilly, K.B. (2019). E-prescribing controlled substances: Here's why the clicks add up. American Medical Association. Retrieved from https://www.ama-assn.org/practice-management/digital/e-prescribing-controlled-substances-here-s-why-clicks-add. (Accessed 7 September 2020.)

Philpot, L.M., Ramar, P., Elrashidi, M.Y., et al. (2017). Controlled substance agreements for opioids in a primary care practice. *Journal of Pharmaceutical Policy and Practice*, 10(1), 29.

Pottie, K., Thompson, W., Davies, S., et al. (2018). Deprescribing benzodiazepine receptor agonists: Evidence-based clinical practice guideline. *Canadian Family Physician*, 64(5), 339–351.

Quinones, S. (2015). Dreamland: The true tale of America's opiate epidemic. London: Bloomsbury Publishing.

Rager, J.B., & Schwartz, P.H. (2017). Defending opioid treatment agreements: disclosure, not promises. *Hastings Center Report*, 47(3), 24–33.

Schuckit, M.A. (2016). Treatment of opioid-use disorders. *New England Journal of Medicine*, 375(4), 357–368.

Shiffman, M.L. (2018). The next wave of hepatitis C virus: the epidemic of intravenous drug use. *Liver International*, 38, 34–39.

St. Marie, B. (2019). Assessing patients' risk for opioid use disorder. *AACN Advanced Critical Care*, 30(4), 343–352.

Stanos, S., Brodsky, M., Argoff, C., et al. (2016). Rethinking chronic pain in a primary care setting. *Postgraduate Medicine*, 128(5), 502–515.

Substance Abuse and Mental Health Services Administration. (2015). *Federal guidelines for opioid treatment programs*. HHS Publication No. (SMA) PEP 15 – FEDGUIDEOTP. Rockville, MD: SAMHSA.

Substance Abuse and Mental eHealth Services Administration. (2018). Medications for opioid use disorder: For healthcare and addiction professionals, policymakers, patients, and families. Retrieved from https://www.ncbi.nlm.nih.gov/books/nbk535275/. (Accessed 7 September 2020.)

Substance Abuse and Mental Health Services Administration. (2020). Apply for a practitioner waiver. Rockville, MD: SAMHSA.

Tobin, D.G., Keough Forte, K., & Johnson McGee, S. (2016). Breaking the pain contract: a better controlled-substance agreement for patients on chronic opioid therapy. *Cleveland Clinic Journal of Medicine*, 83(11), 827–835.

Turner, J.A., Saunders, K., Shortreed, S.M., et al. (2014). Chronic opioid therapy urine drug testing in primary care: prevalence and predictors of aberrant results. *Journal of General Internal Medicine*, 29(12), 1663–1671.

US Department of Health and Human Services. (2019a). HHS guide for clinicians on the appropriate dosage reduction or discontinuation of long-term opioid analgesics. Retrieved from https://www.hhs.gov/opioids/sites/default/files/2019-10/dosage_reduction_discontinuation.pdf. (Accessed 7 September 2020.)

US Department of Health and Human Services. (2019b). Pain management best practices inter-agency task force report: Updates, gaps, inconsistencies, and recommendations. Retrieved from https://www.hhs.gov/ash/advisory-committees/pain/reports/index.html. (Accessed 7 September 2020.)

Verhagen, A.P., Downie, A., Popal, N., et al. (2016). Red flags presented in current low back pain guidelines: a review. *European Spine Journal*, 25(9), 2788–2802.

Veterans Health Administration/Department of Defense. (2017). VA/DoD clinical practice guidelines. Management of opioid therapy (OT) for chronic pain. Retrieved from https://www.healthquality.va.gov/guidelines/pain/cot/. (Accessed 7 September 2020.)

Veterans Health Administration/Department of Defense. (2020). VA/DoD clinical practice guidelines. Retrieved from https://www.healthquality.va.gov. (Accessed 7 September 2020.)

Villaseñor, S., & Piscotty, R.J., Jr. (2016). The current state of e-prescribing: Implications for advanced practice registered nurses. *Journal of the American Association of Nurse Practitioners*, 28(1), 54–61.

Washington State Agency Medical Directors Group. (2015a). Interagency guideline on prescribing opioids for pain, 3rd ed. Retrieved from http://www.agencymeddirectors.wa.gov/files/2015amdgopioidguideline.pdf. (Accessed 7 September 2020)

Washington State Agency Medical Directors Group. (2015b). Opioid dose calculator. Retrieved from https://agencymeddirectors.wa.gov/opioiddosing.asp. (Accessed 7 September 2020.)

Washington State Health Care Authority. (2019). Fast facts for prescribers. Apple Health (Medicaid) opioid policy changes. Retrieved from https://www.hca.wa.gov/assets/billers-and-providers/prescriber-opioids-faq.pdf. (Accessed 7 September 2020.)

Webster, L.R. (2017). Risk factors for opioid-use disorder and overdose. *Anesthesia & Analgesia*, 125(5), 1741–1748.

Wilens, T.E., & Kaminski, T.A. (2020). Stimulants: friend or foe? (Editorial) *Journal of the American Academy of Child and Adolescent Psychiatry*, 59(1), 36–37.

Wilkerson, R.G., Kim, H.K., Windsor, T.A., & Mareiniss, D.P. (2016). The opioid epidemic in the United States. *Emergency Medicine Clinics*, 34(2), e1–e23.

Wolraich, M.L., Hagan, J.F., Allan, C., et al. (2019). Clinical practice guideline for the diagnosis, evaluation, and treatment of attention-deficit/hyperactivity disorder in children and adolescents. *Pediatrics*, 144(4), e20192528.

Legal Aspects of Prescribing 8

Carolyn Dolan

This chapter reviews key legal information to enable advanced practice registered nurses (APRNs) to avoid missteps with the prescriber role. Exemplars are provided to highlight the role of four legal entities that can each play a role in APRN prescribing, particularly if problems occur: Boards of Nursing, malpractice attorneys (if a lawsuit is filed), the Drug Enforcement Administration, and government auditors who monitor nursing facilities. Federal and state prescribing laws are discussed, key issues in safe prescribing are outlined, and risk management strategies are emphasized.

WHAT DO ADVANCED PRACTICE REGISTERED NURSE (APRN) PRESCRIBERS NEED TO KNOW ABOUT THE LAW?

First, APRNs need to know what authority they have under state law and the state's legal requirements for prescribing. Second, they need to know the federal laws on prescribing controlled substances. Third, they need to know the standard of care for prescribing the classes of drugs they intend to prescribe. And fourth they need to know that thousands of APRNs have been able to comfortably navigate the occasional challenges involved with the prescription of medications to help patients improve their health.

APRN prescribing demands practice decisions that are "mindful" and in compliance with all the legal, ethical, and professional expectations that compose the standard of care. Questions of malpractice or unprofessional conduct are broad terms defined by individual state boards of nursing (BONs). If the issue of malpractice related to prescribing occurs, courts of law will look to regulatory, professional, and community criteria to determine the standard of care. The Latin legal maxim "ignorantia juris non excusat" ("ignorance of the law is no excuse") serves as a foundational legal principle that influences the attitudes of governing boards (Law Dictionary, 2019). Although arduous, the APRN's "duty" is to at all times remain knowledgeable about the elements that constitute safe and legal prescribing as well as the current community standard of care. The APRN is individually, professionally, and legally accountable for each and every clinical decision made.

The Advanced Practice Registered Nurse as a Prescriber, Second Edition. Edited by Louise Kaplan and Marie Annette Brown.
© 2021 John Wiley & Sons Ltd. Published 2021 by John Wiley & Sons Ltd.

The license to prescribe is dependent upon a current, unencumbered license to practice. The privilege to prescribe opioids is further delineated by the state Nurse Practice Act (NPA) and federal regulations. Prescribing medication is a significant measure of autonomy that has undergone dramatic change over the past five decades since the inception of the nurse practitioner (NP) role. Certified nurse midwives (CNMs), clinical nurse specialists (CNSs), and certified registered nurse anesthetists (CRNAs) have also been affected by the evolution of prescriptive authority. Medications are usually vital to the patient's individualized plan of care and it is necessary to provide this therapeutic to patients. Prescribing skills are a "touchstone" for APRN best practice. NPs and CNMs prescribe legend drugs in all states, while CRNAs and CNSs have prescribing authority in many but not all states (National Council of State Boards of Nursing [NCSBN], 2020a).

Review of real-world exemplars can provide a "teachable moment," particularly for novice prescribers. The situations that follow have resulted in legal action against APRNs. In addition to peer review by colleagues, there are four entities that have the authority to scrutinize prescribing practices of APRNs. These are BONs, malpractice attorneys if a lawsuit is filed, the Drug Enforcement Administration (DEA) when controlled substances are involved, and government auditors who monitor nursing facilities. This chapter provides examples of cases that resulted in actions against APRNs by each of these entities. These examples reflect actual cases or are taken from BON websites. Box 8.1 contains definitions of terms associated with licensure and potential action on an APRN's license.

CASES INVOLVING BOARDS OF NURSING

States regulate health professions including advanced nursing practice through legislative actions that create Nurse Practice Acts (NPAs). States enact NPAs and delegate the responsibility for their enforcement to BONs. The primary mission of the BON is protection of the public and prevention of harm through the regulation of nursing education, licensure, and practice. Administrative law governs the BON functions of investigative and judicial processes in most nursing licensure matters.

BONs have the legal responsibility to investigate APRNs who are reported for incompetence or unprofessional conduct. Reports may come from nurses, other healthcare professionals, employers, patients, or families. If a board's investigation confirms that an APRN deviated from the standard of care or that an APRN acted unprofessionally, the board may discipline the APRN. Discipline may include a "letter of education" which describes the incident that is placed in the nurse's file but is not accessible to the public. Other types of discipline include a fine, probation, a suspended license, or revocation of a license. The nurse has a property right to the license and the state cannot revoke it without due process. The board also might restrict the nurse's practice, for example, prohibit a nurse midwife from performing deliveries, require continuing education, or require a preceptor to review the APRN's practice decisions that may include activities that involve medication. The following examples highlight situations in which NPs were required to defend themselves before BONs and the lessons learned.

Box 8.1 Terminology

APRN Consensus Model provides guidance for states to adopt uniformity in the regulation of APRN roles (APRN Consensus Work Group, 2008).

Collaborative Practice Agreement (CPA) is a formal legal arrangement with a physician or an NP mentor necessary in some states for advanced practice. It may limit one or more elements of APRN practice (American Association of Nurse Practitioners, 2019).

Competent is defined as "the quality or state of possessing sufficient knowledge, judgment, skill or strength for a particular duty," while "competency" refers to an outcome or measure of adequacy. A key measure of competency for APRNs is national certification (Merriam-Webster, 2020a).

Credentialing is a formal process by which pre-established guidelines are utilized to determine whether a provider is qualified to practice in a specific setting (Merriam-Webster, 2020b).

Disciplinary action refers to step(s) taken by a BON that address an infraction or complaint against the NP.

Encumbered license is a license with current discipline, conditions, or restrictions.

Jurisdiction is the state or territory that a BON regulates (NCSBN, 2020b).

Full practice authority occurs in states with laws that authorize an APRN to evaluate patients; diagnose, order, and interpret diagnostic tests; and initiate and manage treatment that includes the ability to prescribe medication under the sole authority of the exclusive licensing authority of the state BON (American Association of Nurse Practitioners, 2019).

Nurse Practice Act (NPA) details the laws and rules that outline the majority of regulatory requirements for nursing practice through the state BON.

Nursys QuickConfirm License Verification© is a national database for verification of nurse licensure, discipline, and practice privileges for Registered Nurses, Licensed Practical Nurses/Vocational Nurses, and APRNs in participating jurisdictions (NCSBN, 2020b; Nursys, n.d.).

National Practitioner Databank (NPDB) is a repository of reports that contain information on medical malpractice payments and certain adverse events. The agency was established to track practitioners who move from state-to-state without disclosure or discovery of previous damaging conduct (NPDB, n.d.).

Reinstatement is defined as the reissuance of a license following disciplinary action.

Scope of practice (SOP) describes the services an APRN is authorized to perform and undertake under the terms of the professional license.

Unencumbered license indicates that the licensee has full and unrestricted privileges (NCSBN, 2020b).

NP prescribing inconsistent with standard of care

- Case #1 – A BON charged an NP with incompetence after the NP prescribed Synthroid® for a patient without a diagnosis of hypothyroidism. The NP intended to increase the appetite of the patient, an elderly woman who lived in a nursing home. The NP claimed she discussed this unusual therapeutic approach with her collaborating physician who concurred. However, she did not document this discussion. A nursing home auditor identified the NP's activities and reported her to the BON.

- Case #2 – An NP prescribed an extremely large amount of a controlled medication to a man who subsequently sold the pills to a high-school student. The student unintentionally overdosed and died. As part of a criminal investigation, the NP was reported to the BON for failure to practice according to the standard of care. The NP had not documented an adequate assessment, ongoing monitoring, or a rationale for the large number of pills.
- Case #3 – An NP ordered renal function tests in preparation for renal imaging. The radiologist injected the IV contrast prior to the NP or the radiologist's review of the results and the patient suffered renal failure and died. A jury found in favor of the plaintiff's family and awarded $1.7 million in damages.

Lessons learned

APRNs are responsible for practice that is within the standard of care which is to prescribe a medication for an appropriate indication and at an appropriate dose. Accepted dosage ranges may be found in drug reference books and databases commonly used by APRNs. These include Epocrates®, Physicians Drug Reference, and Lexicomp, among others. In the first case, there was no clinical indication for Synthroid®. Trial of an unusual treatment for anorexia could be considered with documentation of evidence to support the effectiveness for her proposed course of treatment. Prescription of "off-label" medications may not be included in the state's NPA and could result in "breach of the standard of care." In the second case, if the NP thought it necessary to prescribe large amounts of a controlled medication, the NP should have documented the rationale for that decision. In the third case, the lack of review and follow-up about the lab results indicated that the NP failed to monitor the patient properly and a jury determined negligence.

NP failed to respond to the effect of prescribed medications

An NP prescribed Coumadin® and ordered international normalized ratio (INR) testing every two weeks but did not adjust the Coumadin dose in response to results. The patient's INR was at non-therapeutic levels for several months. An auditor for Medicaid reported the NP to the BON, and the NP was charged with incompetence.

Lesson learned

NPs are responsible for practicing within the standard of care that includes responding appropriately to laboratory results. In this case, the NP should have increased the dosage of Coumadin® after the test results revealed that the patient was not adequately anticoagulated. Anticoagulants are often indicated in serious medical conditions such as stroke, transient ischemic attack, deep vein thrombosis, and myocardial infarction. They are among the most dangerous prescribed medications due to the risk of adverse events, particularly hemorrhage.

Incumbent upon the prescriber of any medication is the obligation to conduct appropriate monitoring which is not limited to lab tests. The duty extends to monitor the patient and conduct periodic physical examination, update the medical history, assess for drug-to-drug interactions, intolerances, or new allergies. The APRN must update the current medication list at every encounter. All drugs are chemical agents and pose a risk of an untoward effect. The Addictions Center has identified the top fifteen most dangerous drugs or drug classes in order of safety risks as: acetaminophen, alcohol, benzodiazepines, anticoagulants, antidepressants, antihypertensives, bromocriptine, clarithromycin, clozapine, cocaine, colchicine, cough medications, digoxin, heroin, and semisynthetic opioids (e.g. hydrocodone, and oxycodone) (Hilliard, 2019).

NP prescribed for self or family
An NP prescribed a small amount of anti-anxiety medication for herself. A pharmacist reported her to the BON and she was investigated. Another NP prescribed a controlled analgesic for her husband for an episode of back pain. A pharmacist reported the NP to the BON and to her employer. The employer fired the NP, and the BON investigated.

Lesson learned
APRNs are never authorized to prescribe controlled substances for themselves or relatives. Pharmacists and licensing boards are likely to assume that the APRN is self-medicating. Should a pharmacist identify that the patient and prescriber are related, he/she is obligated to report the irregularity to the prescriber's licensing board. APRNs who prescribe a controlled substance for a patient with the same last name might avoid unnecessary reports by a note on the prescription "patient not related to clinician" or by a conversation with the pharmacist.

NP prescribed outside of legal authority
An NP prescribed a Schedule II medication when NPs in the state were authorized to prescribe only Schedules III–V. The BON disciplined the NP. Another NP who did not have DEA registration prescribed a controlled substance because her physician collaborator agreed to "cover her." A pharmacist reported the NP to the BON, who investigated and disciplined the NP.

Lesson learned
State law specifies the controlled substances that NPs may prescribe. NPs may not prescribe outside of that authority. Only NPs with DEA registration may prescribe controlled substances. If a patient requires a medication that the APRN is unable to prescribe, alternative procedures could be used such as referral to or consultation with an appropriate colleague with authority to write the prescription.

CASES INVOLVING CONSULTATION WITH ATTORNEYS
If a medical mishap occurs and a patient suffers an injury, the patient may sue the clinician and the clinician's employer for malpractice. Malpractice (medical negligence) is a civil claim that seeks to hold the APRN legally responsible for

actions that result in an adverse treatment outcome. Examples include failure to inform the patient of the risk/benefit ratio of non-steroidal anti-inflammatory drugs (NSAIDs), failure to monitor renal function properly when prescribing an NSAID, and a subsequent bad outcome linked to these actions (e.g. renal damage). Medication errors and medical judgment mistakes, even when non-intentional, may result in liability. There are four elements that define medical negligence, also known as malpractice:

1. The clinician owed the patient a duty of care
2. The clinician breached the standard of care
3. There was an injury
4. The injury was caused by the breach of the standard of care

For the patient (known as a plaintiff) to mount a successful malpractice case, the patient must prove all four elements (Brous, 2019a, 2019b, 2019c, 2019d, 2019e).

In a lawsuit, both the plaintiff attorney and the defense attorney examine the clinical records related to the patient's care to determine whether the claim has merit. The standard of care is defined in common law (case law) as that degree of care and diligence exercised by a reasonably prudent clinician (e.g. nurse midwife) of similar education and training. To determine the standard of care and whether it was met or breached, both the plaintiff and the defense attorneys rely on the testimonies of expert witnesses. The APRN's defense attorney may argue that one or more of the elements of malpractice were not proven: no duty to the patient was proven; the standard of care was met; there was no injury; or that there was no causal relationship between the breach of the standard of care and the injury.

Criminal charges may be brought in state or federal courts. They can include prescribing a controlled substance without a DEA registration, or other prescribing infractions that fall outside of the APRN's regulatory practice framework, such as failure to follow the CPA or intentional misconduct (diversion). When a criminal case is brought, it follows a process that begins with an investigation and review of information to support specified charges that are then communicated to the accused. A hearing occurs that may produce an indictment, charges, or an arraignment (where a court hearing is scheduled). Next, discovery occurs where both sides gather and review evidence.

Plea-bargaining negotiation may occur prior to the preliminary hearing. If the case is not settled or a disposition reached otherwise, then the case goes to trial. Trials do not always require a jury and in some cases only a judge or a panel of judges is required. After the court hears the case, a verdict is rendered. The last step, the sentence, is also known as the penalty phase. In criminal court, restitution involves the offender who relinquishes freedom (imprisonment) as well as probation or monetary fees. In a criminal case, the losing party may appeal. In a civil case (e.g. malpractice/negligence) either party may appeal the decision. Criminal cases are reported to BONs where licensure discipline occurs. The examples that follow highlight situations in which NPs were required to defend themselves against malpractice claims in civil court and the lessons learned.

NP prescribed without legal authority and appropriate monitoring

A hospital-based NP dramatically increased pain medication dosages for a postoperative patient. The patient had a history of medication abuse and was on methadone as well as analgesics. Nurses had asked the NP to increase the analgesics as the patient's pain was poorly controlled. Shortly after the NP increased the medication dosages, the patient went into respiratory arrest. The patient was resuscitated but sued the hospital and the NP and claimed his cognitive status was impaired after the arrest. The patient's attorneys claimed that the dosages prescribed by the NP were not within the standard of care; the NP failed to properly monitor the patient; and the NP did not have the legal authority to prescribe the medications. The incident occurred in Virginia where an NP may perform functions within the practice of medicine if a physician delegates the authority. The NP stated that she had prescribed under the authority of an anesthesiologist at the hospital. However, the anesthesiologist did not recall authorizing the prescription. At the time of this case, NPs in Virginia did not have the legal authority to prescribe Schedule II medications. The plaintiff won damages of over $1 million.

Lesson learned

The APRN must have the legal authority to prescribe. State laws specify if prescriptive authority includes legend drugs (drugs that require a prescription), controlled substances, or both. State law also regulates which controlled substances may be prescribed and under what circumstances. In the Virginia case, NPs may "practice medicine" if a physician delegates his or her authority. In this case, the NP stated the anesthesiologist at the hospital delegated his authority, which he later denied.

If an attorney can argue effectively against the NP that there was no legal authority to prescribe, then a judge or jury is likely to find that the NP automatically breached the standard of care. In some cases, unprofessional conduct may also be claimed because the NP failed to follow the state's regulations for advanced practice. In this case, the NP's actions would have been more easily defended if the NP documented the delegated authority in the medical record. The NP was not authorized by state law to prescribe Schedule II medications. Furthermore, the NP increased the dosages of analgesics to a threshold where continuous monitoring was indicated but not ordered. The plaintiff's attorney likely argued that this failure to provide the standard of care resulted in the patient's respiratory arrest. NPs must meet the clinical standard of care and must have the legal authority to provide any services rendered.

CASES INVOLVING THE DEA

The DEA is the federal agency charged with enforcement of the Controlled Substances Act (CSA) which governs the manufacture, distribution, prescribing, and possession of controlled substances. Pharmacists or other individuals who suspect that an unauthorized health professional is prescribing controlled substances may report the clinician to the DEA. The DEA will investigate and, if necessary, prosecute the clinician through the US Office of the Attorney General. The following is a case in which an NP was investigated by the DEA.

NP prescribed without DEA registration
A recently graduated NP without DEA registration prescribed a Schedule II medication and did not realize it was a controlled substance. A pharmacist reported her to the DEA; agents arrived at her office and interrogated her. The DEA ultimately decided not to press charges, but her employer was embarrassed by her error and the DEA visit and fired her.

Lesson learned
APRNs who prescribe controlled substances must have DEA registration and prescribe only those schedules allowed by their state law. NPs without a DEA registration must be knowledgeable about whether a medication they intend to prescribe is controlled. Therefore APRNs should consult an up-to-date list of scheduled drugs prior to prescribing. Electronic medication programs such as Epocrates® include such information. The DEA provides a list of controlled substances and pharmacists can be consulted (US Food and Drug Administration, 2020).

Ordinarily, federal laws provide the highest legal authority. However, states may enact laws that are more restrictive than federal law. They cannot, however, weaken federal law. This legal principle is known as preemption. For example, for public safety reasons, some states regulate a medication as a controlled substance, even if it is not under the federal law. One example is the medication gabapentin which in Michigan is a Schedule V drug. In such a case, the APRN must adhere to the laws of the state in which they practice in addition to federal laws.

CASES INVOLVING GOVERNMENT AUDITORS
Nursing facilities must comply with the US Department of Health and Human Services Medicare and Medicaid Conditions of Participation. Periodically, Medicare and Medicaid send auditors into nursing facilities to determine whether federal and state standards are met. Auditors review patient records as one component of the evaluation. If an auditor believes a facility clinician has not met the standard of care, the clinician is reported to the appropriate licensing board. The following case highlights a situation in which an auditor reported the NP.

NP failed to document a verbal order
An NP employed at a nursing facility gave a verbal order to a nurse to discontinue a medication but did not document the order in the record. An auditor for Medicaid reviewed the record and noticed that the orders were not consistent with the care plan. The auditor reported the NP to the BON. The board investigated and charged the NP with incompetence.

Lesson learned
Most facilities have procedures for verbal orders. Generally, the clinician who orders the medication must cosign the order within 24 hours. In this case, the NP should have documented the order to discontinue the medication in the medical record.

SUMMARY

The cases reviewed to this point emphasize the APRN's legal authority to prescribe and the duty to meet the standard of care of a reasonably prudent APRN in a similar setting. There are a variety of ways that APRNs who practice outside of their legal authority or who do not adhere to the standard of care may be identified and reported to regulatory and law enforcement agencies. Therefore APRNs must remain knowledgeable of both the legal parameters of prescribing and clinical standards that define best practice. Legal parameters include:

- Which medications the NP has the legal authority to prescribe under state law
- Which medications are controlled and subject to state and federal regulation
- Limitations on clinician prescribing
- Compliance with requirements associated with opioid prescribing
- Requirements associated with correcting a prescribing error

Clinical standards include:

- An accepted indication for each medication prescribed
- Correct dosage, route, duration, and amount
- Special considerations when prescribing controlled substances for pain
- Monitoring and follow-up of a prescription

The APRN who prescribes a medication must ensure each prescription conforms to all requirements of state and federal laws and regulations. The prescription must meet the standard of care for the condition it is intended to treat.

PUBLIC ACCESS TO LICENSURE STATUS, AND BOARD AND CIVIL ACTIONS

Licensure status and BON actions are public information. BONs use a variety of methods to communicate their information, such as newsletters, databases, and websites. Licensure information and board action for most states are available to the public via Nursys free of charge. License restrictions may occur across a broad spectrum of circumstances – from unintentional mistakes to serious violations that result in harm. Unintentional circumstances could be failure to renew one's license in a timely manner, failure to comply with continuing education requirements, or failure to repay one's student loan. More serious issues might include impairment due to substance use disorder, driving under the influence, malpractice that results in patient harm, and willful, criminal acts. Federal law requires that adverse actions taken against a healthcare professional's license by the individual state are reported to the National Practitioner Data Bank (US Department of Health & Human Services, n.d.).

FEDERAL PRESCRIBING LAWS

Federal prescribing laws focus on controlled substances which are regulated by the CSA. A controlled substance is a drug or chemical substance whose possession and use are regulated under the CSA. The DEA has the authority to enforce the CSA and works in tandem with state agencies to protect the public.

The CSA categorizes controlled substances into five Schedules, I–V, based on the agent's potential for abuse. Although marijuana is a Schedule I agent under the CSA, many states have passed laws for its medical and recreational use. Agents may be removed, added, or changed in the Schedule, usually for public health/safety concerns. For example, hydrocodone was changed from Schedule III to Schedule II in 2014. A special consideration is that the salts, esters, ethers, isomers, and isomer salts and other derivatives of controlled substances may also be controlled substances under the law.

Who may prescribe controlled substances?

APRNs who are authorized by state law, registered with the DEA, and meet any additional state requirements may prescribe controlled substances. The DEA's *Practitioner's Manual* (DEA, 2010) provides essential information, with details of federal requirements for prescribing controlled substances. The process for a prescriber to obtain DEA registration, the purpose of the prescription, the form of the prescription, and how refills may be ordered are specified by federal regulations.

Purpose of a controlled substance prescription

According to the DEA, a prescription for a controlled substance, to be valid, must be issued for a legitimate medical purpose by a practitioner who acts in the usual course of professional practice. According to the CSA, an order purporting to be a prescription not issued in the usual course of professional treatment or as part of legitimate and authorized research is not a valid prescription. The person who knowingly fills an invalid prescription and the person who writes it are subject to penalties.

An individual practitioner may not write a prescription for controlled substances with the intention of supplying the practitioner with controlled substances to dispense to patients. The DEA *Practitioner's Manual* states "A prescription is an order for medication which is dispensed to or for an ultimate user. A prescription is not an order for medication which is dispensed for immediate administration to the ultimate user (for example, an order to dispense a drug to an inpatient for immediate administration in a hospital is not a prescription)."

Form of prescription

According to the DEA *Practitioner's Manual*, a prescription for a controlled substance must be dated and signed on the date when it is written. Federal law prohibits the pre-signing of prescriptions (Code of Federal Regulations – 21 CFR §1306.05, n.d.). If the prescription is not to be dispensed until a date in the future, that should be noted on the prescription as well. The prescription must include the patient's full name and address and the practitioner's full name, address, and DEA registration number. The prescription must also include:

- Drug name
- Strength
- Dosage form

- Quantity prescribed
- Directions for use
- Number of refills (if any) authorized

A prescription for a controlled substance must be written in ink or indelible pencil, typewritten or electronically by a certified digital signature. The prescription must be manually signed by the practitioner on the date when issued or when electronically transmitted. A practitioner may designate an individual (e.g. a nurse or medical assistant) who may prepare a prescription for the practitioner's signature; however, the practitioner is responsible for the accuracy of the prescription.

Electronic prescribing

The DEA adopted rules for electronic prescriptions for controlled substances (EPCS) in 2010 (Controlled Substances Act, Title 21, Part 1311, 2010). The ECPS regulations enable practitioners to write prescriptions for controlled substances electronically. In order to utilize EPCS, a secured system must exist between the prescriber and the destination pharmacy. Specific technology requirements must be established for the pharmacy or pharmacist to receive, dispense, archive, and audit electronic prescriptions. In most states, EPCS is voluntary. Due to the many advantages of EPCS, several states require its use, while others have begun implementation of EPCS. Due to safety benefits for the patient, prescriber, and pharmacist such as decreased diversion, less altering of the prescription, theft, and potential for abuse, EPCS is a significant intervention against opioid abuse and a public health safety feature. Box 8.2 describes the advantages of EPCS for the prescriber, pharmacist, and third parties (auditor, investigator). It is important to note that practitioners are still permitted to communicate Schedule III, IV, and V prescriptions by phone, by fax, or in written form.

Restrictions on amounts prescribed

There is no federal restriction that limits the amount of medication prescribed, although some states and health plans do specify limits. An APRN who prescribes extremely large doses or quantities of controlled substances may come to the attention of the DEA or a BON and may be investigated and disciplined. The investigators may assume that the APRN is careless or diverting drugs. APRNs who have a legitimate reason to prescribe large amounts should carefully document their rationale in the patient's medical record.

Special rules for Schedule II substances

The DEA's *Practitioner's Manual* contains specific rules that pertain only to prescribing Schedule II controlled substances. They require a prescription that must be signed by the practitioner. In an emergency, a practitioner may provide a prescription for a Schedule II controlled substance via telephone. The pharmacist may dispense the prescription if the amount is appropriate for the emergency period. The prescriber must provide a written and signed prescription to the pharmacist within seven days. The pharmacist must notify the DEA if the prescription is not received.

Box 8.2 Ten advantages of EPCS

1. The prescription is reviewed by other professionals and reduces the chance of error.
2. Ease of prescribing for the clinician and receipt and dispensing for the pharmacist when there is secure technology that includes:
   A. Secured entry,
   B. Identity proof
   C. Logical access control.
3. Scheduled II–V drugs may be prescribed electronically. The system allows authorization, authentication, and audit capabilities.
4. Patient's formulary is available and the system can suggest substitutions.
5. Capacity to interface with the state's PDMP.
6. Eliminates issues of illegibility of prescription details.
7. Decreases time spent on prescribing manually.
8. Supports collaborative communication between prescriber and pharmacist.
9. Decreases patient's wait times.
10. Decreases fraud and abuse.

There is no federal expiration date for a Schedule II prescription; states, however, may have time limits. For example, a Schedule II prescription in Washington is valid for one year while a similar prescription in Oregon is valid for two years. There are no federal limits to the quantity of pills dispensed on one prescription. However, some states and many insurance companies limit the quantity dispensed to a 30-day supply. One way the APRN may want to limit the quantity dispensed is to specify on the prescription the length of time it must last, such as 30 days.

There are no refills allowed for a Schedule II controlled substance. There are situations, however, when an APRN may choose to prescribe a controlled substance for use for a few months in the future, which requires a different mechanism than authorization of a refill. While this decision needs to be considered very carefully, a common example is for Ritalin® for a student who will be away at college. The legal mechanism is to use the date in August when the prescriptions are written, and indicate "Do not fill until [ENTER DATE]" with the appropriate date in September and October. Specifically, the DEA's *Practitioner's Manual* (DEA, 2010) says:

> An individual practitioner may issue multiple prescriptions that authorize the patient to receive a total of up to a 90-day supply of a Schedule II controlled substance provided certain conditions are met.

- Each separate prescription is issued for a legitimate medical purpose by an individual practitioner acting in the usual course of professional practice.
- The individual practitioner provides written instructions on each prescription (other than the first prescription), if the prescribing practitioner intends for that prescription to be filled immediately) and indicates the earliest date on which a pharmacy may fill each prescription.

- The individual practitioner concludes that this approach to multiple prescriptions does not create an undue risk of diversion or abuse.
- The issuance of multiple prescriptions is permissible under applicable state laws.
- The individual practitioner complies fully with all other applicable requirements under the CSA and Code of Federal Regulations, as well as any additional requirements under state law.

The DEA's *Practitioner's Manual* warns that its rules should not be construed as encouragement for individual practitioners to issue multiple prescriptions or to evaluate their patients on Schedule II controlled substances less frequently. Caution and sound clinical judgment in accordance with established clinical standards are essential with these practices.

A prescriber may transmit a Schedule II prescription to the pharmacy by facsimile. It cannot be dispensed, however, until the original Schedule II prescription is presented to the pharmacist. Three exceptions to this rule are allowed where the facsimile may serve as the original prescription:

- A practitioner who prescribes a Schedule II controlled substance to be compounded for the direct administration to a patient by parenteral, intravenous, intramuscular, subcutaneous, or intraspinal infusion may transmit the prescription by facsimile. The facsimile prescription is considered a "written prescription" and no further prescription verification is required. All normal requirements of a legal prescription must be followed.
- A practitioner prescribes a Schedule II substance for a resident of a Long Term Care Facility may transmit a prescription by facsimile to the dispensing pharmacy. The practitioner's agent may also transmit the prescription to the pharmacy.
- A practitioner prescribes a Schedule II controlled substance for a patient enrolled in a hospice care program certified and/or paid for by Medicare under Title XVIII or a hospice program that is licensed by the state. The practitioner's agent may also transmit the prescription to the pharmacy. The practitioner or agent should note on the prescription that it is for a hospice patient.

Schedule III–V substances

A practitioner may communicate a prescription for controlled substances in Schedules III–V orally, in writing, by facsimile, or electronically to the pharmacist. An oral prescription must be promptly written by the pharmacist and include all the information required for a valid prescription, except for the signature of the practitioner. The prescription may be refilled if authorized up to five times within six months after the date on which the prescription was issued. After five refills or after six months, whichever occurs first, a new prescription is required.

Prescriptions for Schedules III–V controlled substances may be transmitted by facsimile from the practitioner or an employee or agent of the individual practitioner to the dispensing pharmacy. The facsimile is considered to be equivalent to an original prescription.

Delivery of a controlled substance to persons outside the United States
Controlled substances that are dispensed pursuant to a legitimate prescription may not be delivered or shipped to individuals in another country. Any such delivery or shipment is a prohibited export under federal law.

How to avoid problems as a prescriber of controlled substances
Thousands of health professionals prescribe controlled substances carefully and successfully without difficulties. Very few controlled substances are prescribed for patients without a legitimate need. Consequently, relatively few health professionals are investigated by state boards and the DEA. At the same time, an APRN inevitably assumes some risks when prescribing controlled substances. Possible risks are diversion by the patient, and patient claims that an inappropriate prescription contributed to the development of an addiction; it is also possible that the APRN may become known as a source of controlled drugs in the community. A pharmacist may report the APRN to the licensing board and the DEA if the dosages or amounts prescribed are inappropriately high. Even though the dosages or amounts may be correct, APRNs will be expected to provide rationale for their prescribing decisions.

The risk of patients' diversion can be worrisome for providers because it is impossible to control a patient's behavior. APRNs should be extremely vigilant and meet the DEA and BON's expectations to carefully screen and courageously refuse high-risk patients. While the DEA does not provide guidance to identify these individuals, there are effective strategies that indicate a prescriber has made reasonable efforts to prevent diversion. These include:

- Requiring periodic urine drug screens of patients taking opioids
- Using face-to-face interviews rather than telephone or e-mail to evaluate patients
- Obtaining prior health records and history
- Inquiring about prior experience with recreational drugs
- Documenting all of the precautions noted above

Because of the risk of inadvertent mistakes in complex situations, APRNs are strongly advised to consider referral to a pain specialist for patients with chronic non-cancer pain when one or more of the following situations exist:

- The patient's pain is not well controlled
- Multiple symptoms require management
- The patient cannot perform self-care, and caregivers are inconsistent, strained, or burned out
- The clinician suspects medication abuse triggered by a patient act that deviates from the provider–patient agreement or a urine drug test
- The patient has a history of medication misuse
- There are psychiatric diagnoses or symptoms

Patient referral is one way to illustrate collaboration with experts and explore all available measures to ensure patient safety and to prevent misuse, abuse, overdose, and/or diversion. Responsible prescribers constantly evaluate the effectiveness of their plan, document their evaluations, and make necessary changes with every patient encounter related to controlled substances. Their ongoing surveillance maximizes safe and appropriate care.

Follow-up visits should include evaluation of:

- Analgesia (rating of effectiveness on a scale of 0–10) compared with prior visit
- Ability to perform activities of daily living such as driving, cooking, walking the dog
- A patient who takes controlled substances and drives may present a risk to self or others. Routine assessment and counseling includes advice not to drive in a compromised state. For example, a physician was found liable for failure to warn a patient taking multiple medications not to drive after the patient hit and fatally injured a young boy
- Adverse effects
- Aberrant drug-related behaviors such as requests for early refills

An insightful and informed approach to avoid problems as a prescriber is to be mindful of common mistakes made by other clinicians who prescribe controlled substances. Bolen, an experienced malpractice attorney, outlines common risky errors (Wilner, 2008):

- Failure to respond to patient behaviors
- Poor documentation of referrals
- Failure to justify continued use of pain medication
- Increase in pain medication without rationale
- Use of a benzodiazepine plus opioids without a documented rationale

The DEA has specific indicators to identify providers who inappropriately prescribe. These may include the following:

- The clinician prescribed an inordinately large quantity of controlled substances
- The clinician issued large numbers of prescriptions for controlled substances
- No physical examination was documented
- The clinician warned the patient to fill prescriptions at different pharmacies
- The clinician issued multiple prescriptions to a patient

If an APRN violates prescribing laws, typically an investigation will occur first by state authorities under administrative law. The DEA may conduct its own investigation. If found guilty, the state may revoke the APRN's license and the DEA may request voluntary surrender of the prescriber's DEA registration. Serious abuse and/or diversion violations may invoke federal criminal investigations.

Record-keeping requirements

The DEA's *Practitioner's Manual* specifies requirements for record-keeping for clinicians who prescribe, dispense, and administer controlled substances. It is necessary to record scheduled drugs if they are dispensed at the practice site.

There is no requirement to keep records of controlled substances that are administered. However, practitioners who regularly dispense or administer controlled substances and charge patients a fee for the substances, separately or together with other professional services, must also keep records.

Each practitioner must maintain inventories and records of controlled substances listed as Schedule II, and these must be separate from all other records maintained by the registrant. Likewise, inventories and records of controlled substances in Schedules III–V must be maintained separate from other records, or in such a form that they are readily retrievable from the ordinary business records of the practitioner. All records related to controlled substances must be maintained and be available for inspection for a minimum of two years.

Scheduled drugs that are prescribed for pharmacy dispensing require only the usual documentation (medication, dose, route, timing, amount, and refills, if any) as part of the lawful course of professional practice. Note, however, that state laws may require that clinicians keep records of controlled substances prescribed or copies of prescriptions.

Disposal of controlled substances
A conscientious practitioner will dispose of out-of-date, damaged, or otherwise unusable or unwanted controlled substances, including samples, and transfer them to a registrant who is authorized to receive such materials. These registrants are referred to as "reverse distributors." The practitioner should contact the local DEA field office for a list of authorized reverse distributors and use the appropriate process and forms.

Requirements regarding prescription pads
As of October 1, 2008, federal law requires the use of tamper-resistant prescription pads for Medicaid fee-for-service patients. More than a dozen states have prescription security laws either for all prescriptions or for controlled substances prescriptions. The federally required security requirements features on tamper-resistant prescription pads prevent:

• Photocopying of a completed or blank prescription
• Erasure or modification
• Counterfeiting

In some states, additional security features may be required.

Prescribing off-label
A medication prescribed for an indication or dose not specified in the drug manufacturer's insert is referred to as prescribing off-label. In this common practice, prescribers should know that the indication is not approved by the Food and Drug Administration (FDA), the clinical population is different, or the doses are outside the recommended range. There is no law against prescribing off-label, but it may trigger suspicion. APRNs who prescribe for children typically prescribe off-label, as few drugs have been tested in children. However,

if an APRN prescribes off-label and the patient is injured and sues, the APRN faces a difficult situation. The presumption about standard of care is that drugs are prescribed in accordance with the manufacturer's label instructions. Therefore the APRN will need to rebut the presumption that the off-label medication is not within the standard of care. Consequently, prescribers need to carefully weigh the benefits and risks of prescribing off-label and proceed with caution. Discuss with the patient or parent the rationale for the off-label medication, obtain their approval, and document the discussion and agreement. Useful resources to document or provide rationale for decisions to prescribe off-label include scholarly articles, educational materials, and other sources (*Psychiatry* (Edgmont), 2009).

STATE LAWS ON PRESCRIBING
Authority to prescribe
NPs and CNMs in all states, the District of Columbia (DC), and US territories may prescribe, order, or furnish medications; both CRNAs and CNSs may prescribe in 36 states and DC (NCSBN, 2020a). The legal authority for prescribing is defined differently across the states. Some states, such as Ohio, authorize NPs to prescribe medications specified in a formulary. Georgia allows NPs to prescribe if a physician delegates prescriptive authority. In California, NPs may "furnish" medications under "standardized procedures."

Physician involvement
States vary considerably regarding physician involvement with APRN prescribing. APRNs in some states and DC have full practice authority with no physician involvement. In reduced or restricted practice states, such as Pennsylvania (Box 8.3) and Texas respectively, laws usually address whether or not a nurse must prescribe under a written collaborative agreement, delegation documents, protocols, or standardized procedures agreement with a physician, what must appear on the prescription, and which classes of drugs may be prescribed. This exemplar from Texas specifies dimensions of a written Prescriptive Authority Agreement between an APRN and a physician to enable prescribing:

> (20) Prescriptive authority agreement – An agreement entered into by a physician and an APRN or physician assistant through which the physician delegates to the APRN or physician assistant the act of prescribing or ordering a drug or device (Texas Administrative Code, 2020).

Prescribing for self or family members
APRNs should avoid prescribing for family members, unless the family member is enrolled at a practice where the APRN regularly diagnoses and treats patients. Even if the family members are enrolled patients and the practice is not prohibited by the BON, these prescriptions raise serious ethical questions and in general should not occur. They have inherent risks related to lack of objectivity.

Box 8.3 Example of state law authorizing APRN prescribing in Pennsylvania

A CRNP may prescribe and dispense a drug relevant to the area of practice of the CRNP from the following categories if that authorization is documented in the collaborative agreement (unless the drug is limited or excluded under this or another subsection):

(1) Antihistamines.
(2) Anti-infective agents.
(3) Antineoplastic agents, unclassified therapeutic agents, devices, and pharmaceutical aids if originally prescribed by the collaborating physician and approved by the collaborating physician for ongoing therapy.
(4) Autonomic drugs.
(5) Blood formation, coagulation, and anticoagulation drugs, and thrombolytic and antithrombolytic agents.
(6) Cardiovascular drugs.
(7) Central nervous system agents, except that the following drugs are excluded from this category:
  (a) General anesthetics.
  (b) Monoamine oxidase inhibitors.
(8) Contraceptives including foams and devices.
(9) Diagnostic agents.
(10) Disinfectants for agents used on objects other than skin.
(11) Electrolytic, caloric, and water balance.
(12) Enzymes.
(13) Antitussive, expectorants, and mucolytic agents.
(14) Gastrointestinal drugs.
(15) Local anesthetics.
(16) Eye, ear, nose, and throat preparations.
(17) Serums, toxoids, and vaccines.
(18) Skin and mucous membrane agents.
(19) Smooth muscle relaxants.
(20) Vitamins.
(21) Hormones and synthetic substitutes.

A CRNP may not prescribe or dispense a drug from the following categories:
(1) Gold compounds.
(2) Heavy metal antagonists.
(3) Radioactive agents.
(4) Oxytocics.

Restrictions on CRNP prescribing and dispensing practices are as follows:

(1) A CRNP may write a prescription for a Schedule II controlled substance for up to a 72-hour dose. The CRNP shall notify the collaborating physician as soon as possible but in no event longer than 24 hours.
(2) A CRNP may prescribe a Schedule III or IV controlled substance for up to 30 days. The prescription is not subject to refills unless the collaborating physician authorizes refills for that prescription.

A CRNP may not:

(1) Prescribe or dispense a Schedule I controlled substance as defined in Section 4 of the Controlled Substance, Drug, Device and Cosmetic Act (35 P. S. §780-14).
(2) Prescribe or dispense a drug for a use not approved by the United States Food and Drug Administration without approval of the collaborating physician.
(3) Delegate prescriptive authority specifically assigned to the CRNP by the collaborating physician to another healthcare provider.

A prescription blank shall bear the certification number of the CRNP, name of the CRNP in printed format at the top of the blank, and a space for the entry of the DEA registration number, if appropriate. The collaborating physician shall also be identified as required in §16.91 (relating to identifying information on prescriptions and orders for equipment and service).

The CRNP shall document in the patient's medical record the name, amount, and dose of the drug prescribed, the number of refills, the date of the prescription, and the CRNP's name.

Source: Pa. Regs. §21.284, State board of Nursing, Commonwealth of Pennsylvania.

While there may be no law that specifically prohibits an APRN from prescribing legend drugs, such as antibiotics, for family members, there are legal risks involved. APRNs are particularly vulnerable in states that require a collaborative agreement with a physician. Collaborative agreements are specific to a practice setting; therefore the family member must be enrolled as a patient at the APRN's practice setting in order to prescribe. In states where no collaborative agreement is required, an NP who prescribes for a family member is less vulnerable.

Prescribing legend drugs for oneself is also inadvisable. The APRN should consider that this is not likely to be covered under a collaborative agreement. Furthermore, self-prescribing does not provide the APRN a patient experience with the best healthcare possible. Pharmacy laws in many states make it illegal to prescribe controlled substances for family members or self. Kentucky law is an example of a state that provides guidance on this issue. The Kentucky BON is the legal entity that enforces the laws related to the practice of nursing. It does not restrict the ARNP from prescribing to self or family but advises against the practice in the document Advisory Opinion Statement #37 (AOS), updated in June 2019 (Box 8.4).

Even if prescribing for oneself or relatives is not expressly illegal under many state laws, to prescribe a controlled substance for oneself or a family member is always inadvisable. The pharmacist may suspect that the prescriber, rather than the family member, is using the drug personally and make a report to the licensing board. The APRN may then be in the position of having to prove that he or she is not self-administering controlled substances. Furthermore, DEA registration is specific to a practice setting. An APRN who prescribes a controlled substance for a family member who is not a patient in the practice may violate two laws.

Box 8.4 Kentucky advisory opinion on prescribing for self, family and others in a personal relationship

Legend or Non-Scheduled Pharmaceuticals, Diagnostics, and Therapies
It is the advisory opinion of the Kentucky Board of Nursing that Aprns, with prescriptive authority, not treat themselves, family members, or other persons in a personal relationship except:

- For a minor condition or an emergency situation and only when another qualified healthcare professional is not readily available.
- If an APRN or family member is enrolled as a patient at the APRN's practice setting.

When an APRN does provide care to family members or to other persons within a personal relationship, the APRN should ensure that the person advises his or her healthcare provider of the treatment received.

Controlled Substances: Accepted and prevailing standards of care and Kentucky Law KRS 218A.140(3) https://apps.legislature.ky.gov/law/statutes/statute.aspx?id=39528 presuppose a professional relationship between a patient and practitioner when the practitioner is utilizing controlled substances. By definition, a practitioner may never have such a relationship with himself or herself. It is the advisory opinion that an APRN should not self-prescribe nor self-administer controlled substances. Accepted and prevailing standards of care require that a practitioner maintain detached professional judgment when utilizing controlled substances in the treatment of family members. An APRN should only utilize controlled substances when treating an immediate family member in an emergency situation which should be further documented in the patient's record by their healthcare provider.

Formularies

Some state laws list the medications APRNs may prescribe; other state laws have more general language. Ohio's Exclusionary Formulary specifies drugs that may be initiated by the APRN and drugs that may be prescribed only after the collaborating physician has examined the patient or consulted with the APRN. Ohio law specifies an ARPN may not prescribe a drug or device to perform or induce an abortion or a drug or device prohibited by federal or state law. Alabama's standard formulary of legend non-controlled drugs lists the classifications that may be prescribed by NPs and CNMs (Box 8.5) (Alabama Board of Nursing, 2016).

Standard of care and risk management recommendations of prescribing

Every rare and unusual adverse outcome cannot be prevented. Human error guarantees that occasionally a medication mistake will occur. However, the APRN who understands key legal and safety issues and takes routine measures to lessen risk is less vulnerable. Compliance with general principles of best practice in prescribing reduces liability risk and enhances patient safety. The APRN should discuss medication choice(s) and concerns with the patient and other parties involved in the patient's care; consult (pharmacist, physician collaborator if required) when indicated; remain knowledgeable of clinical guidelines; consult the state prescription drug monitoring program (PDMP); recognize potential drug-to-drug interactions; use appropriate patient care interventions

Box 8.5 Alabama CRNP/CNM formulary of drug classifications

All written prescriptions must adhere to the standard, recommended doses of legend drugs, as identified in the *Physicians' Desk Reference* or the product information insert, not to exceed the recommended treatment regimen periods.

Standard Legend Drugs
1. Anti-Infective Agents
2. Birth Control Drugs, Contraceptive Agents, and Devices
3. Cardiovascular Agents
4. Central Nervous System Agents
5. Dermatological Agents
6. Diagnostic Agents
7. Endocrine and Metabolic Agents
8. Expectorants and Cough Preparations
9. Gastrointestinal Agents
10. Hematological Agents, including Antiplatelet and Anticoagulants & Related Agents
11. Local Anesthetics
12. Musculoskeletal Agents
13. Nutrition and Electrolyte Agents
14. Obstetrical and Gynecological Agents, including Hormones
15. Ophthalmic and Otic Agents
16. Oxytocics for **CNM and Women's Health CNRP only**: May be prescribed according to protocols for management of post-partum bleeding, and in concurrent consultation with the physician for augmentation of labor.
17. Prosthetics/Orthotics
18. Pulmonary and Respiratory Agents
19. Renal and Genitourinary Agents
20. Serums, Toxoids, and Vaccines
21. Vitamins

The Specialty Legend Drugs listed below must be given within the scope of the collaborative practice specialty. The initial dose must be prescribed by a physician, with authorization to prescribe continuing maintenance doses according to written protocol (available for review on site) or direct order of the physician. Other requirements are listed below:

Specialty Legend Drugs
1. Antineoplastic Agents
2. Oxytocics
3. Radioactive Agents: *Collaborating physician must have current license from the Alabama Department of Public Health for prescribing and dispensing radioactive pharmaceuticals.*
4. Non-biologic disease-modifying anti-rheumatic drugs (DMARDs)
5. Biologic or Biosimilar DMARDs and Anti-tumor necrosis factor drugs (anti-TNF)
6. Other Biologics or Biosimilars (excluding anti-TNF)

(e.g. patient exams and lab monitoring); and perform regular medication reconciliation. An inadvertent omission such as the failure to update a new drug allergy can be life-threatening. Good stewardship, especially discontinuation of medications no longer indicated, and constant vigilance of medications that pose a greater risk than benefit (e.g. a NSAID in a patient with decreased renal function or recalled medication) all demonstrate due diligence as a prescriber.

The availability of malpractice insurance is an important safeguard for APRNs. Nurses Service Organization (NSO) is the nation's largest provider of nursing malpractice insurance. NSO analyzes professional liability claims against NPs periodically. Data from the five-year period 2011–2016 related to medication management and prescribing are provided in Table 8.1. Medication-related claims represented 29.4% of all closed claims. The overall frequency of medication-related allegations in the report nearly doubled to 16.5% since the 2012 report. The three most frequent medication-related allegation categories against NPs were improper prescribing or management of controlled drugs; failure to recognize contraindications and/or known adverse drug-to-drug interactions; and improper management of medications (CNA and Nurses Service Association, 2017).

Additional principles for safe prescribing include (Buppert, 2020):

- With every prescription, go through a SCRIPT analysis:
  - Side effects – Do I need to alert the patient about what to watch for?
  - Contraindications – Do any listed contraindications pertain to this patient? If so, should I prescribe something else?
  - Right medication, dose, frequency, and route – Have I checked all of these against a reference?
  - Interactions – Might any of the patient's other medications interact with this one? If so, should I prescribe something else?
  - Precautions – Do any listed precautions pertain to this patient? If so, should I prescribe something else?
  - Transmittal – Is my writing legible to others?
- Write no prescription without an appropriate patient evaluation and documentation in the patient's chart.

Table 8.1 Selected frequency and severity of allegations related to medication prescribing

Allegation	Percentage of closed claims with indemnity payment	Average paid indemnity (US$)
Improper prescribing/management of controlled drugs	12.9% highest frequency	99,662
Wrong medication	0.7%	60,000
Wrong dose	2.4%	167,000
Failure to recognize contraindication and/or known adverse interaction between ordered medications	4.3%	461,146
Failure to provide proper medication instructions	1.0% highest severity	795,000

- Refer to a pain specialist for chronic pain disorders not responding to guidelines for opioid prescribing.
- Medical record documentation:
  - Keep the refill record in a central place in the chart, rather than documenting refills only in the note for the daily visit.
  - Record prescriptions transmitted to pharmacies while away from the office.
  - Self-audit your documentation with a critical eye.
- Counsel patients for whom you have prescribed controlled substances that they should not drive, and document the advice.

Additional important questions to consider to reduce risk are:

- Is the prescription absolutely necessary?
- Has the patient received refills of controlled substances only at the appropriate and expected times?
- Am I in compliance with state and federal laws in providing this prescription? This includes licensure, credentialing, and educational requirements.
- Am I consulting the state PDMP periodically or in accordance with regulations?
- Have I followed current guidelines for prescribing controlled substances?
- Have I counseled patients prescribed controlled substances that they should not drive, operate machinery, or attempt technical skills?
- Have I documented the advice given to patients?

LIABILITY INSURANCE

The American Nurses Association (ANA), the American Association of Nurse Practitioners (AANP), and the American Association of Nurse Attorneys (TAANA) strongly recommend that nurses carry their own, individual malpractice and licensure defense insurance. Some APRNs have a misconception that an individual liability policy is not necessary if they are covered by their employer. Employer-based policies have numerous limitations and should supplement not supplant one's own individual coverage. Sometimes institutional power dynamics will influence the APRNs level of protection if multiple providers are involved. Major considerations about employer-based coverage are that, generally, employer-based insurance does not provide license defense protection and will not extend beyond the hours of employment. In other words, should you provide an APRN action "off the clock," for example offering to change a neighbor's dressing or to give an injection, and a subsequent claim of negligence occurs, the employer-based policy would not provide coverage.

It is also important to consider that employer-based insurance may not provide coverage for APRN action(s) if deemed outside of organizational policies and procedures. For example, should the APRN prescribe an off-label medication and there is an adverse outcome, the employer's carrier may determine that the coverage is not in effect for acts inconsistent with organizational policies or accepted treatment guidelines. For example, a policy may state all prescribed medication must be FDA approved for the purpose, indication, and guidelines for use. As professionals, APRNs are urged to carry individual malpractice/licensure protection that is always active.

Types of insurance

There are two basic types of liability policies, but there are also a few key features that the APRN should consider. Generally, policy coverage is either claims-based or occurrence based.

Claims-based or claims-made coverage means that protection is available only for claims that occur while the policy is in effect and are "filed" during the time that the policy is active. Occurrence-based policies provide coverage of any occurrence that happens while the policy is in force, no matter when the claim is filed. Tail coverage is recommended with claims-based policies to provide extended coverage. Tail coverage can be purchased as an addition to the policy if it is not renewed or the APRN leaves the practice setting. For example, an APRN purchases a claims-based policy for a certain practice setting but changes employers. The claims-based coverage ends at termination of employment, but potentially claims against the APRN may still occur. Tail coverage "extends" liability protection for a certain length of time even though the APRN has left the practice setting. The length of time the coverage is in effect is specific to the contract provisions but typically correlates to the statute of limitations for filing a tort claim.

While occurrence-based policies are more expensive, they provide better coverage. A key factor in the decision about the type of coverage is to compare the cost of claims-based coverage plus tail insurance against the cost of occurrence-based. Another core element to consider is the limits of the policy. The contract will specify effective dates as well as limits of amounts. Many are written as $1 million/$3 million or $1 million per claim up to $3 million total amount of coverage per year. Additionally, some organizations "self-insure." The limits of coverage for the APRN under a self-insured agency's policy are contract specific. The APRN will need to know the terms of the coverage.

CONCLUSION

Knowledge of prescribing laws and attention to standards of care are essential for effective and safe prescribing as well as reduced risk. To ensure compliance with prescribing laws and procedures, annual review of the BON website, the Nurse Practice Act, and any additional prescribing regulations enhances APRN safety. In addition, periodic review of the DEA website allows APRNs to remain abreast of changes in federal laws. It is imperative that APRNs sustain their knowledge of laws, regulations, policies, opinions, and advisories regarding prescribing. The critical area of controlled substances requires significant attention to identify new or revised recommendations for prescribing set forth by professional associations or state boards. Although adherence to guidelines is not the only way to demonstrate rational prescribing, it contributes to the maintenance of a high standard of care. Continuing education provides excellent opportunities to remain abreast of current information on medication and prescribing practices.

Information provided in this chapter offers guidance to decrease legal risks and avoid difficult situations. Damage caused from medications, especially from mistakes or poor practice, may be impossible to undo. A patient's legal remedy – monetary damages – never makes the patient whole. Consequences of disciplinary action because of a complaint to the BON can be life-changing for the APRN. Disciplinary processes and litigation exact an emotional cost and may be professionally catastrophic. Human error may occur even when providing high-quality care.

Prevention of errors is well worth the effort. Attention to professional standards as well as state and federal laws significantly increases APRN confidence, competence, and satisfaction in practice. More importantly, it promotes patient safety. The prescribing role is an essential component of practice and medications may significantly enhance a patient's quality of life. Despite the challenges, experience and careful attention can contribute to the development of a competent APRN prescriber.

DISCLAIMER

The information provided is for educational purposes only and is not to be construed as individual legal advice and does not establish an attorney–client relationship. Individuals with specific legal concerns should consult an attorney with healthcare expertise, e.g. a nurse attorney.

REFERENCES

Alabama Board of Nursing. (2016). Alabama CRNP/CNM formulary of drug classifications. Retrieved from https://www.abn.alabama.gov/wp-content/uploads/2016/05/crnp-cnm-standard-formulary.pdf. (Accessed 7 September 2020.)

American Association of Nurse Practitioners. (2019). State practice environments: practice environment details. Retrieved from https://www.aanp.org/advocacy/state/state-practice-environment. (Accessed 7 September 2020.)

APRN Consensus Work Group. (2008). Consensus model for APRN regulation: Licensure, accreditation, certification & education. Retrieved from https://www.ncsbn.org/consensus_model_for_aprn_regulation_july_2008.pdf. (Accessed 7 September 2020.)

Brous, E. (2019a). The elements of a nursing malpractice case, Part 1: Duty. *American Journal of Nursing*, 119(7), 64–67.

Brous, E. (2019b). The elements of a nursing malpractice case, Part 2: Breach. *American Journal of Nursing*, 119(9), 42–46.

Brous, E. (2019c). The elements of a nursing malpractice case, Part 3A: Causation. *American Journal of Nursing*, 119(11), 54–59.

Brous, E. (2020d). The elements of a nursing malpractice case, Part 3B: Causation. *American Journal of Nursing*, 120(1), 63–66.

Brous, E. (2020e). The elements of a nursing malpractice case, Part 4: Harm. *American Journal of Nursing*, 120(3), 61–64.

Buppert, C. (2020). *Prescribing: Preventing legal pitfalls for NPs*. Bethesda, MD: Law Office of Carolyn Buppert.

CNA and Nurses Service Organization. (2017). Nurse practitioner claim report: 4th Edition. Retrieved from https://aonaffinity-blob-cdn.azureedge.net/

affinitytemplate-dev/media/nso/images/documents/cna_cls_np_101917_ cf_prod_sec.pdf. (Accessed 7 September 2020.)

Code of Federal Regulations – 21 CFR §1306.05. (n.d.) Manner of issuance of prescriptions. Retrieved from https://www.ecfr.gov/cgi-bin/text-idx?SID= 3f78cdacf1325206b5a8b2d44f51a1b0&mc=true&node=se21.9.1306_105&rgn =div8. (Accessed 7 September 2020.)

Controlled Substances Act, Title 21, Part 1311. (2010). Requirements for electronic orders and prescriptions. Retrieved from https://www. deadiversion.usdoj.gov/21cfr/cfr/1311/subpart_c100.htm. (Accessed 7 September 2020.)

Drug Enforcement Administration. (2010). Practitioner's manual. [Under revision.] Retrieved from https://www.deadiversion.usdoj.gov/pubs/index. html. (Accessed 7 September 2020.)

Hilliard, J. (2019). Addiction Center. The top 15 most dangerous drugs. Retrieved from https://www.addictioncenter.com/news/2019/08/15-most-dangerous-drugs/. (Accessed 7 September 2020.)

Law Dictionary. (2019). Ignorantia juris non excusat. Retrieved from https:// dictionary.thelaw.com/ignorance-of-the-law/. (Accessed 7 September 2020.)

Merriam-Webster. (2020a). Competence. Retrieved from https://www.merriam-webster.com/dictionary/competence. (Accessed 7 September 2020.)

Merriam-Webster. (2020b). Credential. Retrieved from https://www.merriam-webster.com/dictionary/credentialing. (Accessed 7 September 2020.)

National Council of State Boards of Nursing. (2020a). Member board profiles: 2019 advanced practice registered nurse survey. Retrieved from https:// www.ncsbn.org/2019aprn.pdf. (Accessed 7 September 2020.)

National Council of State Boards of Nursing. (2020b). Nursys. Retrieved from https://www.nursys.com. (Accessed 7 September 2020.)

National Practitioner Data Bank (n.d.) About us. Retrieved from https://www. npdb.hrsa.gov/topnavigation/aboutus.jsp. (Accessed 7 September 2020.)

Nursys. (n.d.). Nursys glossary of terms. Retrieved from https://www.nursys. com/help/glossary.aspx#r. (Accessed 7 September 2020.)

Psychiatry (Edgmont). (2009). Liability and off-label prescriptions. Psychiatry, 6(2), 43–44.

Texas Administrative Code. (2020). §§ 22.1 and 222.2. Advanced practice registered nurses with prescriptive authority. Retrieved from http://txrules. elaws.us/rule/title22_chapter222_sec.222.2. (Accessed 7 September 2020.)

US Department of Health and Human Services. (n.d.) National Practitioner Data Bank. Retrieved from https://www.npdb.hrsa.gov/. (Accessed 7 September 2020.)

US Food and Drug Administration. (2020). Approved drug products with therapeutic equivalence evaluations (orange book). Retrieved from https:// www.fda.gov/drugs/drug-approvals-and-databases/approved-drug-products-therapeutic-equivalence-evaluations-orange-book. (Accessed 7 September 2020.)

Wilner, A.N. (2008). Medico-legal aspects of managing pain. Medscape Neurology. Retrieved from https://www.medscape.org/viewarticle/581931. (Accessed 7 September 2020.)

Medical Marijuana and the APRN

9

Louise Kaplan

Legalization of marijuana continues to occur worldwide and in many US states and jurisdictions. In some of the states, one or more of the APRN roles may provide patients with authorizations to use medical marijuana. This chapter offers an overview of marijuana as a drug, federal and state law, the typical process to provide an authorization, standards of care, and the evidence-base for medical marijuana.

Countries around the world have fully or partially legalized medical and recreational marijuana; others have made cannabis-derived products available for medical use. Some have decriminalized recreational marijuana or made its use and possession legal but not its sale. An APRN needs to know the policies, best practices, and evidence-base for medical marijuana. An APRN may be able to legally authorize medical marijuana, patients may ask advice about marijuana use for their problems, friends will ask for an opinion about marijuana use, and there are circumstances in which marijuana use is contraindicated. This chapter provides an overview of medical marijuana laws, types of marijuana products, the process for providing authorizations to qualifying patients, and the evidence-base for medical marijuana use.

DEFINITIONS

As marijuana and cannabis are often used interchangeably in policy and science, both terms will be used in this chapter.

- Cannabidiol (CBD) is a cannabinoid that acts on cannabinoid receptors, has no psychoactive effects, and may attenuate the psychoactive effects caused by tetrahydrocannabinol (THC).
- THC is the cannabinoid responsible for the psychoactive effects of marijuana.

The Advanced Practice Registered Nurse as a Prescriber, Second Edition. Edited by Louise Kaplan and Marie Annette Brown.
© 2021 John Wiley & Sons Ltd. Published 2021 by John Wiley & Sons Ltd.

- *Cannabis* is the proper botanical name for the plant, while marijuana is the term associated with the use of the plant. Typically there is reference to two major strains, *sativa* and *indica*.
- Medical marijuana is legalized for use by patients with qualifying health conditions when authorized by a healthcare professional.
- Recreational marijuana refers to all other uses of the substance, including non-authorized use for a health condition.

PHARMACOLOGY

Marijuana is derived from the cannabis plant. The plant contains more than 100 cannabinoids of delta-9-tetrahydrocannabinol (THC) which have psychoactive effects. Evidence for their potential therapeutic benefit will be discussed later in the chapter. Marijuana products may be used as a combination of THC and CBD, while there are also CBD-only products, some of which may be sold without a prescription.

Although marijuana is a Schedule I controlled substance in the US, there are legal synthetic THC and CBD medications administered orally. Dronabinol, a Schedule III drug, is a THC product indicated for the treatment of anorexia associated with weight loss in people with acquired immunodeficiency syndrome (AIDS) as well as nausea and vomiting associated with cancer chemotherapy for people who do not respond to other antiemetic treatment (UNIMED Pharmaceuticals, 2004). Nabilone, a Schedule II drug, is a synthetic cannabinoid product also indicated for nausea and vomiting associated with cancer chemotherapy in people who failed to respond to other antiemetic treatment (Valeant Pharmaceuticals International, 2006). Epidiolex is a legal CBD legend drug approved for the treatment of seizures associated with Lennox-Gastaut or Dravet syndrome in people two years of age or older (Greenwich Biosciences, 2020).

People who use medical marijuana may choose one or more of several methods of administration, although state law will guide whether each is considered legal. Prescribed products, such as nabilone, are administered orally. Marijuana may be smoked and vaporized. Dabbing is a superheated form of vaporization of oils or waxy extracts of cannabis. Foods and drinks may be infused with cannabis, referred to as edibles. Sativex is a prescription cannabis medication available only in Europe that uses oromucosal administration.

Marijuana produces euphoria, sedation, and hallucinations, which no other drug is capable of doing (Rosenthal & Burchum, 2018). When inhaled, about 60% of the THC content is absorbed. Onset of the effects occurs within minutes and last two to three hours. When ingested, activation occurs on first pass through the liver; therefore higher doses are required for oral use than when inhaled. Generally the ingested form has a delayed onset of 30–50 minutes and the effect may last up to 12 hours (Rosenthal & Burchum, 2018).

Marijuana can cause short-term adverse effects. A person may develop cardiovascular symptoms such as tachycardia and hypotension; neurological effects including dizziness, headaches, disorientation, and sleepiness; respiratory symptoms such as cough, bronchodilation, and wheezing; and psychiatric symptoms including anxiety, paranoid thinking, apathy, and hallucinations (Natural Medicines, 2020).

Long-term side effects may also occur. There is substantial evidence of an association between maternal cannabis smoking and lower birth weight in newborns. Moderate evidence supports an association between regular cannabis use and increased symptoms of mania and hypomania in individuals with bipolar disorders, an increased incidence of suicide completion, and an increased incidence of social anxiety disorder (National Academies of Sciences, Engineering, and Medicine [NASEM], 2017). Cannabis use disorder, cannabinoid hyperemesis syndrome, and cannabis withdrawal syndrome are additional potential long-term consequences of regular and/or problematic cannabis use (American Psychiatric Association, 2013; Freeman & Winstock, 2015; Lu & Agito, 2015).

There is limited research regarding drug–drug interactions; nonetheless, the possibility needs to be considered. Cannabis may depress the central nervous system (CNS) and interact with other CNS depressants, and may prolong bleeding time when people use warfarin (LexiComp, 2020).

LEGALIZATION

Canada and Uruguay have fully legalized marijuana for recreational and medical use. Many more countries have legalized medical marijuana such as Argentina, the Czech Republic, Germany, Greece, Israel, Malawi, the Netherlands, Portugal, Switzerland, Thailand, and Zimbabwe (Wikipedia, 2020). In the United States, marijuana is illegal under federal law; however, 36 states, the District of Columbia (DC), Guam, Puerto Rico, and the US Virgin Islands have legalized comprehensive medical marijuana programs (National Conference of State Legislatures [NCSL], 2020). Recreational marijuana is legal for adults in 15 states, DC, and the Northern Mariana Islands (NCSL, 2019).

People who use marijuana

Data reveal a changing picture of the ages of people who use marijuana. The US National Survey on Drug Use and Health collected data between 2015 and 2018 that indicate cannabis use among adults aged 65 and older increased from 2.4% to 4.2% (Han & Palamar, 2020). A 2017 National Poll on Healthy Aging surveyed adults aged 50–80 about marijuana use for medical purposes. Six percent of respondents reported medical marijuana use and 44% would definitely consider asking a healthcare provider about marijuana if they had a serious health condition that might respond to its use (University of Michigan, 2018). Among adolescents in grades 8, 10, and 12 (typically ages 13 to 18) who participated in a national survey in 2017, marijuana use had a combined prevalence (all three grades) of 23.9%. This was a significant increase of 1.3% from the prior year, although daily marijuana use changed little (Johnston et al., 2018).

In 2018 there were an estimated 2,132,777 medical marijuana patients in the United States (ProCon.org, 2018). Not all states require patients to be entered into a registry and not all states with registries report numbers. Consequently, this estimate likely underrepresents the number of medical marijuana patients. Canada had 369,614 medical client registrations in September 2019 (Canada Health, 2019). Germany introduced medical marijuana in March 2017; by the end of 2019, there were 10,255 people approved for medical marijuana use, while 47,331 people had their application rejected, mainly because they did not have documented use of alternative therapies that are required prior to application (Medical Cannabis Network, 2020). Israel first permitted medical use of marijuana in the 1990s for people with cancer and certain pain-related conditions. In 2019, Israel had an estimated 38,000 medical marijuana patients (Lidman, 2019).

Support for marijuana legalization

The American Legion has openly advocated for safe access, quality products, and investment in research for veterans. The American Legion is a non-profit service organization whose members are veterans of the US military. Many veterans experience the physical, emotional, and social costs of traumatic brain injury and post-traumatic stress disorder (PTSD). The American Legion (2016) adopted a resolution in 2016 that urged the Drug Enforcement Administration (DEA) to license privately funded medical marijuana production operations to enable safe and efficient cannabis drug development research. The resolution also urged Congress to remove marijuana from Schedule I and reclassify it to acknowledge its potential medical value.

Although illegal at the federal level, Rep. Earl Blumenauer (D-OR) founded a Congressional Cannabis Caucus in 2017. It is intended to serve as a forum for members of the US House of Representatives to work together to develop a more rational approach to federal cannabis policy. It has bipartisan leadership and membership (Baretto, 2019).

Public support for marijuana use and policy reform has increased. A 2019 Pew Research Center survey revealed that two-thirds of Americans supported the legalization of marijuana for both medical and recreational use. Another 32% support legalization of marijuana for medical use. Combined, 91% support some form of marijuana legalization (Daniller, 2019).

US federal law

Marijuana is a DEA Schedule I drug as listed in the Controlled Substances Act of 1970, a category for drugs with high potential for abuse, no accepted medical use, and a lack of accepted safety (DEA, 2017). Other Schedule I drugs include heroin, lysergic acid diethylamide, and methylenedioxymethampehatime (ecstasy). Enforcement of the federal law is discretionary. Under President Barack Obama's administration, the Department of Justice 2013 Guidance on Marijuana Enforcement established eight priorities and emphasized prevention of distribution to minors and sales that are a cover for trafficking or cartels. The guidance discouraged prosecution of non-violent users of marijuana and indicated there would be no interference in states with laws that regulate marijuana use, sales, and distribution if the safety of the public is protected (Cole, 2013). In 2018, this guidance was rescinded by President Donald Trump's administration (Sessions, 2018).

The Agricultural Improvement Act of 2018 (the 2018 Farm Bill) removed hemp, derived from the *Cannabis sativa* plant, from the Controlled Substance Act when there is no more than 0.3% THC contained in the product. The 2018 Farm Bill maintained the US Food and Drug Administration's (FDA) authority to regulate cannabis or cannabis-derived products under the Food, Drug, and Cosmetic Act (FDA, 2020b). THC and CBD products are both excluded from the definition of a dietary supplement. Sale of CBD products purportedly with less than 0.3% THC is widespread, with many producers making unfounded health claims. The FDA monitors sales, many of which are web-based, and issues warning letters (FDA, 2020b). State legalization of these CBD products creates another patchwork of regulatory approaches to cannabis products.

As a Schedule I controlled substance, marijuana research is subject to a highly regulated process which makes it slow and onerous. Application to conduct clinical research is made to the FDA's Center for Drug Evaluation and Research. If an application is approved, site-specific DEA registration must be obtained. Marijuana must be supplied through the National Institute on Drug Abuse Drug Supply Program that requires another review process (FDA, 2020a). There is, however, some federal support for CBD and cannabinoid research. In the fiscal year 2019, the National Institutes of Health (NIH) awarded $220 million to researchers for the investigation of a variety of topics, especially pain (NIH, 2020).

US state laws
Although legalized in US jurisdictions, the federal designation as a Schedule I controlled substance makes it illegal to prescribe. Consequently, in the jurisdictions that have legalized medical marijuana, healthcare professionals do not prescribe marijuana but instead authorize, recommend, or certify (subsequently referred to as authorize) an individual to use medical marijuana. The individual receives an authorization, recommendation, and certificate of referral (hereafter referred to as authorization) used to obtain marijuana products. Additional states have laws that allow limited access to low THC/high CBD products, often in the context of research studies or without permitting in-state production, making access to out-of-state products for dispensaries or individuals difficult or impossible (NCSL, 2020).

State laws vary widely regarding who can provide a medical marijuana authorization, what conditions qualify a patient for medical marijuana use, and the processes required to determine if a patient has a qualifying condition. In DC, Hawaii, New Hampshire, Minnesota, New Mexico, and Washington, all APRNs may provide medical marijuana authorizations. In Maine, Massachusetts, New York, and Vermont, nurse practitioners (NPs) are permitted to provide authorizations. Colorado allows NPs who have earned prescriptive authority to provide authorizations for disabling, but not debilitating, conditions. Each state has established a medical marijuana program to regulate patient access to and use of medical marijuana.

AUTHORIZATIONS
Requirements to provide authorization
In many states there are no special requirements necessary for a healthcare provider to qualify to provide medical marijuana authorizations. Some states, such as Florida and New York, require completion of an education course. Another requirement is that the provider must register and create an account with the

state through which authorizations are submitted (e.g. Colorado, Massachusetts, Minnesota, and New York).

Requirements about the patient–provider relationship

Some states require the patient and healthcare provider to have an established relationship prior to the medical marijuana request. Washington State law requires the provider to have a documented relationship as the principal care provider or specialist who is responsible to monitor and treat the patient's terminal or debilitating condition. Several states stipulate there be a "bona fide healthcare professional–patient relationship" (e.g. Colorado, Hawaii, Maine, Massachusetts, and Vermont). Vermont requires that the patient–provider relationship has been established at least three months unless the patient has a terminal illness, cancer, or AIDS, or is in hospice care (Vermont Department of Public Safety, 2020).

Qualifying conditions

Each state determines which conditions qualify a patient to receive a medical marijuana authorization. There are dozens of qualifying conditions among the different states; some conditions are more commonly designated than others. Typically, the conditions must be debilitating, intractable, or terminal, or the person has not responded to standard treatment. Common conditions include cachexia, cancer, Crohn's disease, epilepsy, glaucoma, hepatitis C, human immunodeficiency virus (HIV)/AIDS, nausea, chronic pain, and multiple sclerosis (Russell et al., 2018).

Depression is not a qualifying condition in any state, although New Jersey, Pennsylvania, and West Virginia have designated anxiety as a qualifying condition. Depression and anxiety have been reported as the two most common psychiatric reasons that regular marijuana users consume marijuana without a healthcare professional authorization (Osborn et al., 2015). New York, New Jersey, and Pennsylvania include opioid use disorder as a qualifying condition. In some states such as California, the healthcare provider may decide if marijuana use will provide relief for a condition not specified as qualifying, or they may petition a designated group. Effective December 2018, Maine eliminated all qualifying conditions, therefore allowing access to a medical marijuana certification for any reason (Maine Department of Administrative and Financial Services, 2020). Table 9.1 lists the qualifying conditions for medical marijuana in each of the states in which an APRN may provide the authorization.

Screening prior to authorization

It is important to consider special populations and circumstances when a medical marijuana authorization may not be appropriate even if the person has a qualifying condition. Certain groups are more vulnerable to the potential adverse effects of marijuana. There also may be little or no reliable evidence that demonstrates an association between marijuana and health outcomes in the population (NASEM, 2017). These groups include adolescents and young adults, pregnant women, neonates, children being breastfed, older adults, and people with certain mental health problems such as schizophrenia or psychotic conditions.

Table 9.1 Qualifying conditions in states in which one or more APRN role can provide medical marijuana authorizations

Condition	Colorado[1]	District of Columbia[2]	Hawaii[3]	Massachusetts[4]	Minnesota[5]	New Hampshire[6]	New Mexico[7]	New York[8]	Vermont[9]	Washington[10]
Amyotrophic lateral sclerosis (ALS)	x	x		x	x	x		x		
Alzheimer's disease	x				x	x	x			
Arthritis (rheumatoid)			x				x			
Autism spectrum disorder	x				x		x			
Cachexia	x	x	x	x		x	x	x	x	x
Cancer	x	x	x	x	x	x	x	x	x	x
Chronic/intractable pain			x	x	x	x	x	x	x	x
Crohn's disease/inflammatory bowel disease		x		x	x	x	x	x	x	x
Epilepsy/seizures	x	x	x	x	x	x	x	x	x	x
Glaucoma	x	x	x	x	x	x	x	x	x	x
Hepatitis C				x		x	x			x
HIV/AIDS	x	x	x	x		x	x	x	x	x
Multiple sclerosis	x	x	x	x	x		x	x	x	x
Nausea		x	x	x		x	x	x	x	x
Neuropathies							x	x		
Parkinson's disease				x		x	x	x	x	
Persistent muscle spasms	x	x	x	x	x	x		x		x

(Continued)

Table 9.1 (Continued)

Condition	Colorado[1]	District of Columbia[2]	Hawaii[3]	Massachusetts[4]	Minnesota[5]	New Hampshire[6]	New Mexico[7]	New York[8]	Vermont[9]	Washington[10]
PTSD	x	x	x		x	x	x	x	x	x
Spinal cord injury						x	x	x	x	x
Others	Any condition for which a physician could prescribe an opioid	Chemotherapy and radiation therapy using azidothymidine or protease inhibitors Decompensated cirrhosis	Lupus Conditions approved by the director of Department of Health or designee	Other debilitating conditions as determined by the healthcare provider	Sleep apnea Terminal illness	Muscular dystrophy Chronic pancreatitis Lupus Ehlers-Danlos syndrome	Friedrich's ataxia Hospice care Inclusion body myositis Lewy body disease Obstructive sleep apnea Opioid use disorder Spasmodic torticollis Spinal muscular atrophy Patient may petition	Huntington's disease Substance use disorder		Traumatic brain injury

[1] https://www.colorado.gov/pacific/cdphe/recommend-medical-marijuana
[2] https://medicalmarijuana.procon.org/legal-medical-marijuana-states-and-dc/ (ProCon.org, 2020)
[3] https://www.capitol.hawaii.gov/hrscurrent/vol06_ch0321-0344/hrs0329/hrs_0329-0121.htm
[4] https://www.mass.gov/doc/guidance-for-health-care-providers-on-the-medical-use-of-marijuana/download
[5] https://www.health.state.mn.us/people/cannabis/patients/conditions.html
[6] https://www.dhhs.nh.gov/oos/tcp/medical-conditions.htm
[7] https://www.nmhealth.org/about/mcp/svcs/hpp/
[8] https://regs.health.ny.gov/content/section-10042-practitioner-issuance-certification
[9] https://medicalmarijuana.vermont.gov/medical-and-mental-health-professionals
[10] https://app.leg.wa.gov/rcw/default.aspx?cite=69.51a.010

Determination if woman may be pregnant or breastfeeding should be standard practice to allow for appropriate counseling and shared decision making. In Florida, physicians must document whether a woman is pregnant and pregnant women may only receive authorization for low THC cannabis (Florida Statutes, 2019). While not always stipulated in law, providers are encouraged to screen patients for past or current substance misuse or the presence of mental health problems which may be exacerbated by marijuana use. Also consider whether a urine drug screen may be beneficial.

Providing authorization

Some states require in-person evaluation of a patient for initial and renewal of medical marijuana authorization (e.g. Colorado, New Hampshire). Others allow follow-up care or renewal to be via telehealth after an initial in-person visit (e.g. Hawaii, Minnesota, and New Mexico). There are considerable ethical issues involved with authorizing medical marijuana for oneself or a member of one's family. Massachusetts explicitly prohibits a healthcare provider from issuing an authorization for oneself or immediate family member for medical marijuana (Cannabis Control Commission, 2017).

Regulations often differ for patients under the age of 18 years. In Colorado, Florida, and Massachusetts, two providers must concur that a minor qualifies for the use of medical marijuana, one of whom must be a pediatrician (Cannabis Control Commission, 2017; Colorado Department of Public Health & Environment, 2019; Florida Statutes, 2019). Typically, the patient's parent/guardian will need to provide informed consent. New Mexico requires a copy of the minor's birth certificate.

States also stipulate the type of documentation required for submission to the medical marijuana program. This may be print or electronic. Once entered into a registry, the patient is eligible to purchase marijuana at a store or dispensary. In almost all states, patient entry into a registry is mandatory and provides some legal protection for the patient.

The APRN is also advised to determine if the encounter for a medical marijuana authorization will be covered by insurance. Washington State law indicates health plans are not required to provide reimbursement for claims related to the medical use of marijuana (Washington State Legislature, 2019). In contrast, New York does require health plans to reimburse for an office visit if the service is a covered benefit and also resulted in a medical marijuana authorization (Johnson, 2017). Minnesota law specifies that neither medical assistance nor MinnesotaCare, a healthcare program for Minnesotans with low income, can reimburse an enrollee or provider for the costs associated with the medical use of marijuana (2019 Minnesota Statutes, 2019a).

Patient evaluation

Provision of an authorization for the medical use of marijuana for a terminal, debilitating, or disabling condition requires a comprehensive evaluation. In the situation when a patient has received ongoing care from the APRN, the evaluation may differ from the situation in which a patient presents to establish care and requests a medical marijuana authorization. Elements of the evaluation should include a history of the illness, past history, social history, family history, and screening for mental health conditions and substance use, and for women whether pregnancy or breastfeeding is present. It is important to include and document therapies that have been used to treat the condition without adequate therapeutic response. A comprehensive physical examination, review of supporting documents from other healthcare professionals such as chart notes, laboratory tests, and diagnostic examinations, and a diagnosis complete the evaluation.

Informed and shared decision making

The decision to provide a medical marijuana authorization requires the APRN to offer information about the risks and benefits of marijuana as well as the evidence-base for its use. Options for methods of administration, particularly for the marijuana naïve patient, approaches to dosing, side effects, necessary restrictions such as not operating motor vehicles or heavy equipment when using marijuana, and what to expect as a response to marijuana use are critical information to discuss.

Shared decision making starts with asking the patient "What matters to you?" and "What is the matter?" (Barry & Edgman-Levitan, 2012). More than 20 years ago, four essential characteristics of shared decision making were identified and remain highly relevant to current practice (Charles et al., 1997):

1. At a minimum, the clinician and patient are involved in the treatment decision-making process.
2. Both the clinician and patient share information with each other.
3. Both the clinician and patient participate in the decision-making process by expressing preferred treatments.
4. Both the clinician and patient agree to the treatment.

The decision to proceed with a medical marijuana authorization may be made at the initial encounter or at a subsequent office visit to allow the patient to consider the information and evidence. Once the patient is ready, a joint decision should result in a treatment plan. If the patient is a minor or does not have decision-making capacity, parent, guardian, or surrogate involvement is required.

Treatment

The Federation of State Medical Boards *Model Guidelines for the Recommendation of Marijuana in Patient Care* (2016) recommends the following elements of a treatment plan.

- Review of other measures attempted to ease the suffering caused by the terminal or debilitating medical condition that do not involve the recommendation of marijuana.
- Advice about other options for managing the terminal or debilitating medical condition.

- Determination that the patient with a terminal or debilitating medical condition may benefit from the recommendation of marijuana.
- Advice about the potential risks of the medical use of marijuana to include:
  o The variability of quality and concentration of marijuana;
  o The risk of cannabis use disorder;
  o Exacerbation of psychotic disorders and adverse cognitive effects for children and young adults;
  o Adverse events, exacerbation of psychotic disorder, adverse cognitive effects for children and young adults, and other risks, including falls or fractures;
  o Use of marijuana during pregnancy or breast feeding;
  o The need to safeguard all marijuana and marijuana-infused products from children and pets or domestic animals; and
  o The need to notify the patient that the marijuana is for the patient's use only and the marijuana should not be donated or otherwise supplied to another individual.
- Additional diagnostic evaluations or other planned treatments.
- A specific duration for the marijuana authorization for a period no longer than twelve months.
- A specific ongoing treatment plan as medically appropriate.

Wilsey et al. (2015) proposed the use of a Medical Cannabis Treatment Agreement for patients who experience chronic pain, similar to one used with patients prescribed opioids. The use of a treatment agreement developed to assure patients are informed of their responsibilities for the safe use of marijuana. The goal is to avoid problems with misuse and abuse of marijuana that occurred when opioids were widely prescribed without opioid treatment agreements. The agreement can be used for patients with authorizations for medical marijuana for any qualifying condition. There are 12 tenets recommended in the model Medical Cannabis Treatment Agreement (Box 9.1).

The treatment plan should include whether medical marijuana will be authorized, whether new medications are prescribed or refills provided, circumstances under which the patient should return for further evaluation, and when follow-up should occur. While a state may require only an annual visit for the patient to renew a medical marijuana authorization, APRNs should consider the need for more frequent follow-up care. Patients with terminal, debilitating, or disabling conditions often benefit from the support and review of their experiences with medical marijuana.

Documentation
The evaluation, treatment plan, and supporting documentation should be part of the patient record. If a cannabis agreement is used, the patient should be provided with a copy and one included in the record, along with the appropriate documentation for the actual medical marijuana authorization. For example, a form must be completed in New Mexico and Washington State that is given to the patient. In some states the APRN will submit the documentation through an online portal.

Box 9.1 Appendix 1 Medicinal Cannabis Agreement

Date:

I understand that (clinician name) is helping me with the treatment of my chronic pain. In considering the possibility of using medicinal cannabis, it is important to recognize that the risks of medicinal cannabis may be impacted by specific medical conditions and patterns of use. I understand what has been explained to me and agree to the following conditions of treatment:

1. I must prevent children and adolescents from gaining access to medicinal cannabis because of potential harm to their well-being. I will store cannabis in locked cabinets to prevent anyone else from using it.
2. I know that some people cannot control their use of cannabis. One example is using cannabis for reasons other than for the indication for which it was prescribed; like getting stoned. This may lead to not going to work, or not doing my household chores. I agree to discuss this with my provider if this happens.
3. I realize that unless specifically recommended by my provider, I should abstain from medicinal cannabis if:
   (a) I am pregnant or am of child-bearing age
   (b) I am middle-aged or older and have a heart disease or heart rhythm problem
   (c) I have a history of serious mental illness (e.g., schizophrenia, mania, or a history of hallucinations or delusions)
4. In order to reduce the risk of lung disease, I will avoid smoking cannabis with tobacco; avoid deep inhalation or breath-holding; and use a vaporizer rather than smoke joints or use a water pipe.
5. I will not drive a car or operate heavy machinery for 3–4 hours after use of medicinal cannabis, or longer if larger doses are used or the effects of impairment persist. I will use a designated driver for automobile transportation if I have to go out sooner than 3–4 hours after taking this medicine.
6. As the potency of cannabis varies widely I will use the minimum amount of medicinal cannabis needed to obtain relief from pain or other symptoms. When trying a new strain of cannabis, I will start with a very small amount and wait at least 10 minutes to see how it affects me.
7. If thought advisable by my health care provider, I might want to substitute one of the Food and Drug Administration (FDA) approved medicines containing THC rather than take natural cannabis.
8. I might notice a withdrawal syndrome for two weeks if I stop cannabis abruptly. Trouble getting to sleep and angry outbursts might require that I withdraw from the cannabis slowly.
9. I understand that the course of treatment will have to be re-evaluated regularly after I start the medicinal cannabis.
10. I will not use medicinal cannabis in public places unless the law specifically permits this.
11. I know there is no legal precedent to help me if I am terminated from employment if a urine toxicology screen is positive for cannabis.
12. I know that I may be asked to reduce or stop my intake of opioids (narcotics), sedative-hypnotics (benzodiazepines), and/or alcohol. This will be done to reduce the risk of side-effects from a combination of medications that affect the central nervous system.

Signed: _____

Source: Modified from Fischer et al., 2011.

Patient education

Some laws specify the patient who uses medical marijuana should be advised about the risks and benefits of the drug. This should be a standard part of informed consent and patient education. It is essential that the APRN counsel women who are pregnant or lactating about the potential effects of marijuana on the fetus or child. Education about the effects of marijuana on the developing brain is a critical element of informed consent for a patient under the age of 18 and in general for any patient under the age of 25 (NASEM, 2017).

Side effects of marijuana's use should be discussed, especially for the marijuana naïve patient. Cannabis use may induce short-term side effects mainly on the CNS, as previously discussed. Patients will also ask about how to use marijuana. Only prescribed cannabis products (dronabinol, nabilone, and epidiolex) will have specific dosing regimens. Marijuana products used for medicinal purposes may be smoked, inhaled, or ingested, although a few states prohibit smoking marijuana, such as Pennsylvania and Louisiana (ProCon.org, 2020). Minnesota allows vaporized delivery of liquid or oil which does not require dried leaves or plant form (2019 Minnesota Statutes, 2019b). If a patient prefers ingestion of marijuana product, it is important to explain that the effects of the drug may be delayed pending digestion and absorption. As patients self-titrate, emphasize the principle of *start low and go slow*. Prepare them that trial and error is necessary to determine the most beneficial administration method, formulation, quantity, and frequency (Russell et al., 2018). Although there are hundreds of strains of marijuana sold in stores, there is no scientific research to guide product selection.

Many people who use marijuana, both medical and recreational, have children. It is imperative to provide education about safety measures to protect children from accidental or recreational use of marijuana. Edibles in the form of cookies, candy, and infused drinks may have particular appeal to a child. In families with older children and teens, ongoing vigilance is necessary for parents and guardians to prevent recreational use of marijuana similar to prescribed controlled substances. Colorado's marijuana program (Colorado Marijuana, 2019) recommends keeping marijuana products in child-resistant packing, clearly labeled, and locked in secure storage.

Sample guidelines

Box 9.2 contains the authorization guidelines for Washington State that includes required and recommended elements of patient evaluation, the treatment plan, ongoing treatment, treatment of minors and people without decision-making capacity, maintenance of health records, and continuing education. This is a comprehensive synthesis of the law and best practices.

Legal issues

It is necessary that APRNs who provide authorizations review and thoroughly understand the requirements of their state's marijuana law. State laws typically provide legal protection for the healthcare professional from criminal liability if they provide advice and an authorization. Other members of the team such as registered nurses or medical assistants may not have this protection, as is the

---

Box 9.2 Authorization practice guidelines from Washington State

A healthcare practitioner may provide valid documentation to authorize medical marijuana (cannabis) to a qualifying patient under Chapter 69.51A RCW under the following conditions:

SECTION 1: PATIENT EVALUATION

A healthcare practitioner should obtain, evaluate, and document the patient's health history and physical examination in the health record prior to treating for a terminal or debilitating condition.

(a) The patient's health history should include:
   i. Current and past treatments for the terminal or debilitating condition;
   ii. Comorbidities; and
   iii. Any history of substance misuse or abuse using a risk assessment tool.
(b) The healthcare practitioner should:
   i. Complete an initial physical examination as appropriate based on the patient's condition and medical history; and
   ii. Check the Prescription Drug Monitoring Program database for the patient's receipt of controlled substances.
   iii. Review the patient's medications including indication(s), date, type, dosage, and quantity prescribed.
   iv. Provide the qualifying patient and their designated provider (if any) each with a medical marijuana authorization form printed on tamper-resistant paper containing the RCW 69.51A.030 logo as required under WAC 246-71-010.

SECTION 2: TREATMENT PLAN

A healthcare practitioner should document a written treatment plan that includes:
(a) Review of other measures attempted to treat the terminal or debilitating medical condition that do not involve the medical use of marijuana;
(b) Advice about other options for treating the terminal or debilitating medical condition;
(c) Determination that the patient may benefit from treatment of the terminal or debilitating medical condition with medical use of marijuana;
(d) Advice about the potential risks of the medical use of marijuana to include: The variability of quality and concentration of medical marijuana:
   i. Adverse events, including falls or fractures;
   ii. The unknown short-term and long-term effects in minors, as more fully explained in Section 4, below;
   iii. Use of marijuana during pregnancy or breast feeding; and
   iv. The need to safeguard all marijuana and marijuana-infused products from children and pets or domestic animals;
   v. Additional diagnostic evaluations or other planned treatments;

(e) A specific duration for the medical marijuana authorization for a period no longer than 12 months for adults (age 18 and over) and 6 months for minors (under age 18); and
(f) A specific ongoing treatment plan as medically appropriate.

SECTION 3: ONGOING TREATMENT

A healthcare practitioner should conduct ongoing treatment and assessment as medically appropriate to review the course of the patient's treatment, to include:

(a) Any change in the medical condition;
(b) Any change in physical or psychosocial function;
(c) Any new information about the patient's terminal or debilitating medical condition; and
(e) An authorization may be renewed upon completion of an in-person physical examination.
(f) Following an in-person physical examination, evaluate patient eligibility for a compassionate care renewal of their authorization per RCW 69.51A.030(2) (c)(iii).

SECTION 4: TREATING MINOR PATIENTS OR PATIENTS WITHOUT DECISION MAKING CAPACITY

The risks of marijuana use in minors are substantial, particularly given its well-documented adverse effects on the developing brain.[1] While research demonstrates that the use of marijuana can be helpful for adults with specific debilitating conditions, there are no published studies on the use of medical marijuana for minors. A healthcare practitioner should strongly consider limiting the authorization of marijuana to minors in palliative pediatric care when short-term symptom relief outweighs long-term risks. The most common symptoms that may justify the use of medical marijuana for minors are pain, nausea, vomiting, seizures, and agitation.[2]

Under RCW 69.51A.220 and RCW 69.51A.230(4), a healthcare practitioner considering authorizing marijuana to a patient under the age of 18 or without decision making capacity must:

(a) Ensure the patient's parent, guardian, or surrogate participates in the treatment and agrees to the medical use of marijuana;
(b) Evaluate and document history of substance misuse or abuse using a risk assessment tool[3];
(c) Consult with other healthcare practitioners involved in the patient's treatment, as medically indicated and as agreed to by the patient's parent, guardian, or surrogate, before authorization or reauthorization of the medical use of marijuana; and
(d) Include a follow-up discussion with the minor's parent or patient surrogate to ensure the parent or patient surrogate continues to participate in the treatment;
(e) Ensure the patient's parent, guardian, or surrogate acts as the designated provider; and
(f) Reexamine the minor at least once every six months or more frequently as medically indicated.

(Continued)

Additional requirements to note when treating minor patients:

(a) Qualifying patients (adult or minor) can only have one designated provider under RCW 69.51A.010. This can be challenging for minor patients who live in divorced families.

(b) School districts must permit a designated provider (parent/legal guardian) to administer marijuana-infused product to a minor qualifying patient (under age 18) in accordance with school policy at the request of a parent – RCW 69.51A.225.

(c) The minor may not grow plants or purchase marijuana (cannabis) – RCW 69.51A.220.

(d) Both the minor and the minor's parent or guardian who is acting as the designated provider must be entered in the medical marijuana authorization database and hold a recognition card – RCW 69.51A.220.

SECTION 5: MAINTENANCE

A healthcare practitioner should maintain the patient's health record in an accessible manner, readily available for review, and include:

13. The diagnosis, treatment plan, and therapeutic objectives;
14. Documentation of the presence of one or more recognized terminal or debilitating medical conditions identified in RCW 69.51A.010(24).
15. Documentation of other measures attempted to treat the terminal or debilitating medical condition that do not involve the medical use of marijuana;
16. A copy of the signed authorization form for both the patient and their designated provider (if any);
17. Results of ongoing treatment; and
18. The healthcare practitioner's instructions to the patient.

SECTION 6: CONTINUING EDUCATION

A healthcare practitioner issuing authorizations or valid documentation for the medical use of marijuana on or after the effective date of these guidelines should complete a minimum of three hours of continuing education related to medical marijuana.

Such program should explain the proper use of marijuana (cannabis), including the pharmacology and effects of marijuana (e.g., distinction between cannabidiol (CBD) and tetrahydrocannabinol (THC); methods of administration; and potential side effects or risks).

[1] https://pediatrics.aappublications.org/content/135/3/584.
[2] The federal Food and Drug Administration (FDA) has approved medications related to marijuana that are available in pharmaceutical grade by prescription for rare conditions. One of the medications is approved for the treatment of seizures associated with Lennox-Gastaut syndrome or Dravet syndrome in patients over two years of age. This medication is not considered medical marijuana and is not available at marijuana dispensaries. This medication is prescribed by subspecialists with expertise in these conditions.
[3] The use of a risk assessment tool is particularly important in the treatment of minors. The American Academy of Pediatrics developed a guide to help providers incorporate screening, brief intervention, and referral for the use of alcohol, tobacco, marijuana, and other drugs among adolescent patients. https://pediatrics.aappublications.org/content/138/1/e20161210.

case in Washington State (Washington State Legislature, 2019). Employers may not be required to make accommodations for an employee who uses medical marijuana, as in New Hampshire (New Hampshire Statutes, 2016). This should be considered if an APRN wants to become a medical marijuana patient. States may prohibit the APRN whose clinical practice includes medical marijuana authorization from any economic interest in a business that produces, processes, or sells medical marijuana or other potential conflicts of interest (Washington State Legislature, 2019).

Reasons why clinicians do not provide authorization
Among respondents to a Washington State survey of healthcare professionals' knowledge, attitudes, and practices, only 18.5% had ever issued a medical marijuana authorization (Kaplan et al., 2019). Participants who did not provide authorizations were asked to indicate the reasons. The most commonly reported reason (58%) was the lack of knowledge and skills necessary to provide authorizations. Over one-third (38%) worked in a practice with a policy that prohibited medical cannabis authorizations, with 21% citing receipt of federal money as the reason for not providing authorizations. Other reasons included concern about medical marijuana use (32%), never had a request (31%), concern about legal problems (22%), concerns about the lack of an evidence base (16%), and other reasons (20%).

THE EVIDENCE BASE FOR MEDICAL MARIJUANA
Policy makers do not always use evidence to make decisions. Medical marijuana qualifying conditions are an example of this. Were evidence used, all states would have the same qualifying conditions. Consequently, it is incumbent upon APRNs to incorporate into shared decision making the science that underpins the use of medical marijuana. Scientific evidence has increased as the legal use expands. Still, many clinicians and the public utilize anecdotal information from the media and on the internet. It is essential to read studies that provide high levels of high-quality evidence. Systematic reviews that assess the overall level and quality of evidence about a topic are especially important to understand whether the evidence is sufficient.

Sources of evidence
Many healthcare professionals are acutely aware of their need for more in-depth knowledge about marijuana. A study of Washington State healthcare professionals (medical and osteopathic physicians, APRNs, physician assistants, and naturopathic physicians) revealed 64% used other healthcare professionals as a source of information, followed by continuing education (47%). Reports from patients and scientific journals were used by 31% of respondents. Other sources of information included websites (22%); medical marijuana consultants (11%), a role unique to Washington State; family and friends (6%); and books (2%) (Kaplan et al., 2019). A Colorado survey of family practice physicians identified medical literature as the most commonly used source of information, followed by experiences with patients, news media, other physicians, lecture, continuing education, friends/family, practice policy, other, and dispensary owners (Kondrad & Reid, 2013). APRNs are urged to use scientific

evidence as the main source of information for themselves and patients to assure the level and quality of the evidence can be assessed.

What is the evidence?

NASEM convened the Committee on the Health Effects of Marijuana: An Evidence Review and Research Agenda to conduct a comprehensive review of the evidence regarding the health effects of using cannabis and cannabis-derived products. In addition to evaluating evidence, research gaps were identified and future research recommendations developed. The report of the committee, *The Health Effects of Cannabis and Cannabinoids: The Current State of the Evidence and Recommendations for Research*, was published in January 2017 (NASEM, 2017). Although more evidence has since been published, the report remains a cornerstone of marijuana research.

The report used five categories of evidence to reach its conclusions regarding cannabis or cannabinoids and their effectiveness when used for therapeutic purposes and whether there is an association with a health endpoint of interest when used for recreational purposes. These categories of evidence are conclusive and substantial; moderate; limited; and no or insufficient. Selected findings of the report are shown in Box 9.3.

As new evidence emerges, APRNs will want to review the study methods, sample size, limitations, bias, and potential confounding factors. Some studies may enroll a small number of participants, for example 10–20, and not have sufficient power to draw conclusions. Studies of the same health condition may not be comparable if different forms of cannabis were used in the research. For example, it is difficult to compare outcomes when one study included cannabis that is smoked, another used cannabis that is vaporized, and another used prescribed nabilone.

Mass-marketed books, industry journals, and websites about marijuana and its effects should be carefully scrutinized. Books written by a healthcare professional about marijuana may or may not be evidence based and caution is necessary for endorsement of its quality. There are many professional and advocacy organizations that promote publications favorable to marijuana's use for medical purposes despite the absence of scientific evidence. Many websites promote different strains of marijuana for different health conditions.

Other than prescribed cannabis-derived medications, there is no standardized testing and evaluation of which commercially sold strains of marijuana would have benefit for specific conditions. Many times claims are made that certain strains are effective for conditions for which no evidence of effectiveness exists. This makes it exceedingly difficult to provide patients with guidance for what marijuana products to use. Despite these issues, APRNs can develop the skills necessary to summarize the current research constraints as well as the state of the science for patients in a neutral but factual way.

Guidelines for APRN practice and education

The National Council of State Boards of Nursing (NCSBN) convened the NCSBN Medical Marijuana Guidelines Committee to produce *The NCSBN National Nursing Guidelines for Medical Marijuana* (Russell et al., 2018), a report and recommendations to assist nurses who provide care to people who use

---

Box 9.3 Selected findings of *The Health Effects of Cannabis and Cannabinoids* report (pp. 13–14)

Conclusive or substantial evidence that cannabis or cannabinoids were effective was found for:

- Treatment of chronic pain in adults
- As antiemetics for people with chemotherapy-induced nausea and vomiting
- For spasticity self-reported by people with multiple sclerosis (MS).

Moderate evidence supported cannabis or cannabinoids were effective for:

- Sleep disturbance associated with obstructive sleep apnea
- Fibromyalgia
- Chronic pain
- Multiple sclerosis.

Limited evidence was found that cannabis or cannabinoids were effective for:

- Increasing appetite and decreasing weight loss in people with HIV/AIDS
- Clinician measured spasticity associated with MS
- Improving symptoms of Tourette syndrome
- Improving symptoms of social anxiety as assessed by a public speaking test
- Improving symptoms of PTSD.

No or insufficient evidence was identified to support or refute the effectiveness of cannabis or cannabinoids as an effective treatment for:

- Cancer
- Cancer-associated anorexia cachexia syndrome and anorexia nervosa
- Symptoms of irritable bowel syndrome
- Epilepsy
- Spasticity in patients with paralysis due to spinal cord injury
- Symptoms associated with amyotrophic lateral sclerosis
- Chorea and certain neuropsychiatric symptoms associated with Huntington's disease
- Motor system symptoms associated with Parkinson's disease or the levodopa-induced dyskinesia
- Dystonia
- Achieving abstinence in the use of addictive substances
- Mental health outcomes in individuals with schizophrenia or schizophreniform psychosis.

---

medical marijuana, education for pre-licensure nursing programs, education for APRN programs, and APRNs who certify patients for medical marijuana use. The report sets forth nine recommendations regarding APRN education (Box 9.4) and six for APRN practice to assure the APRN is appropriately educated and prepared with the principles and knowledge for medical marijuana patient safety (Box 9.5). The recommendations promote evidence-based

---

Box 9.4 NCSBN recommendations for APRN student education

The APRN student shall:

(1) Have a working knowledge of the current state of legalization of medical and recreational cannabis use.
(2) Have working knowledge of the principles of a medical marijuana program.
(3) Have an understanding of the endo-cannabinoid system, cannabinoid receptors, cannabinoids, and the interactions between them.
(4) Have an understanding of cannabis pharmacology and the research associated with the medical use of cannabis.
(5) Shall be able to recognize signs and symptoms of cannabis use disorder and cannabis withdrawal syndrome.
(6) Shall be able to identify the safety considerations for patient use of cannabis.
(7) Shall be aware of medical marijuana administration considerations.
(8) Shall be aware of the ethical considerations related to the care of a patient using medical marijuana.
(9) Shall follow specific employer policies and procedures, terms of the collaborative agreement, standard care arrangement, and facility policy and procedures regarding certifying a qualifying condition.

Box 9.5 NCSBN recommendations for APRN practice

The APRN shall:

(1) Have a working knowledge of the current state of legalization of medical and recreational cannabis use.
(2) Have knowledge of the jurisdiction's medical marijuana program.
(3) Have an understanding of the endocannabinoid system, cannabinoid receptors, cannabinoids, and the interactions between them.
(4) Have an understanding of cannabis pharmacology and the research associated with the medical use of cannabis.
(5) Be able to recognize signs and symptoms of cannabis use disorder and cannabis withdrawal syndrome.
(6) Have an understanding of the safety considerations for patient use of cannabis.

---

practice. Adoption and application of the guidelines in APRN education and practice are strongly recommended.

CONCLUSION

The rapidly changing regulatory landscape of medical marijuana laws and science requires APRNs to be well prepared to respond to questions, give evidence-based advice, and assist patients with decision-making about medical marijuana use. APRNs are not required to provide marijuana authorizations and can thoughtfully choose whether to provide authorizations. If not, referral to another provider is appropriate. Nonetheless, APRNs have a responsibility to promote patient safety and inform patients about the evolving evidence base as well as the need for further research to determine best practices and effectiveness. As always, patients deserve a thoughtful, informed discussion about medical marijuana use, its potential risks, benefits, adverse reactions, and alternatives.

REFERENCES

Minnesota Statutes. (2019a). Chapter 152. Section 152.23: Limitations. Retrieved from https://www.revisor.mn.gov/statutes/cite/152.23. (Accessed 7 September 2020.)

Minnesota Statutes. (2019b). Chapter 152. Section 152.22: Definitions. Retrieved from https://www.revisor.mn.gov/statutes/cite/152.22. (Accessed 7 September 2020.)

American Psychiatric Association. (2013). Diagnostic and Statistical Manual of Mental Disorders, *Fifth Edition*. Washington, DC: American Psychiatric Association.

Baretto, T. (2019). Blumenauer announces co-chairs of Congressional Cannabis Caucus for 116th Congress. Retrieved from https://blumenauer.house.gov/media-center/press-releases/blumenauer-announces-co-chairs-congressional-cannabis-caucus-116th. (Accessed 7 September 2020.)

Barry, M.J., & Edgman-Levitan, S. (2012). Shared decision making – the pinnacle of patient-centered care. *New England Journal of Medicine*, 366(9), 780–781.

Canada Health. (2019). Data on cannabis for medical purposes. Retrieved from https://www.canada.ca/en/health-canada/services/drugs-medication/cannabis/research-data/medical-purpose.html. (Accessed 7 September 2020.)

Cannabis Control Commission. (2017). Guidance for healthcare providers regarding he medical use of marijuana. Retrieved from https://www.mass.gov/doc/guidance-for-health-care-providers-on-the-medical-use-of-marijuana/download. (Accessed 7 September 2020.)

Charles, C., Gafni, A., & Whelan, T. (1997). Shared decision-making in the medical encounter: what does it mean? (or it takes at least two to tango). *Social Science & Medicine*, 44(5), 681–692.

Cole, J.M. (2013). Guidance regarding marijuana enforcement. Retrieved from https://www.justice.gov/iso/opa/resources/3052013829132756857467.pdf. (Accessed 7 September 2020.)

Colorado Department of Public Health & Environment. (2019). Recommend medical marijuana. Retrieved from https://www.colorado.gov/pacific/cdphe/recommend-medical-marijuana. (Accessed 7 September 2020.)

Colorado Marijuana. (2019). Safe storage. Retrieved from https://www.colorado.gov/pacific/marijuana/safe-storage. (Accessed 7 September 2020.)

Daniller, A. (2019). Two-thirds of Americans support marijuana legalization. Pew Research Center. Retrieved from https://www.pewresearch.org/fact-tank/2019/11/14/americans-support-marijuana-legalization/. (Accessed 7 September 2020.)

Drug Enforcement Administration. (2017). Drugs of abuse: A DEA resource guide. Retrieved from https://www.dea.gov/sites/default/files/drug_of_abuse.pdf. (Accessed 7 September 2020.)

Federation of State Medical Boards. (2016). Model guidelines for the recommendation of marijuana in patient care. Retrieved from https://www.fsmb.org/siteassets/advocacy/policies/model-guidelines-for-the-recommendation-of-marijuana-in-patient-care.pdf. (Accessed 7 September 2020.)

Fischer, B., Jeffries, V., Hall, W., et al. (2011). Lower risk cannabis use guidelines for Canada (LRCUG): a narrative review of evidence and recommendations. *Canadian Journal of Public Health*, 102(5):324–327.

Florida Statutes. (2019). Medical use of cannabis. *Chapter 381.986*. Retrieved from http://www.leg.state.fl.us/statutes/index.cfm?app_mode=display_statute&url=0300-0399/0381/sections/0381.986.html. (Accessed 7 September 2020.)

Freeman, T.P., & Winstock, A.R. (2015). Examining the profile of high-potency cannabis and its association with severity of cannabis dependence. *Psychological Medicine*, 45(15), 3181–3189.

Greenwich Biosciences. (2020). Highlights of prescribing information. Retrieved from https://www.epidiolex.com/sites/default/files/pdfs/epidiolex_full_prescribing_information_04_16_2020.pdf. (Accessed 7 September 2020.)

Han, B.H., & Palamar, J.J. (2020). Trends in cannabis use among older adults in the United States, 2015–2018. *JAMA Internal Medicine*, 180(4), 609–611.

Johnson, L. (2017). Health insurance coverage for medical marijuana. *Insurance Circular Letter No. 6*. Retrieved from https://www.dfs.ny.gov/insurance/circltr/2017/cl2017_06.htm. (Accessed 7 September 2020.)

Johnston, L.D., Miech, R.A., O'Malley, P.M., et al. (2018). Monitoring the future national survey results on drug use, 1975–2017: Overview, key findings on adolescent drug use. Ann Arbor: Institute for Social Research, University of Michigan.

Kaplan, L., Klein, T., Wilson, M., & Graves, J. (2019). Knowledge, practices, and attitudes of Washington State health care professionals regarding medical cannabis. *Cannabis and Cannabinoid Research*, 5(2).

Kondrad, E., & Reid, A. (2013). Colorado family physicians' attitudes toward medical marijuana. *Journal of the American Board of Family Medicine*, 26(1), 52–60.

Lexicomp. (2020). Cannabis. Retrieved from https://online.lexi.com/lco/action/login. (Accessed 7 September 2020.)

Lidman, M. (2019). Medical cannabis reform leaves at least 5,000 patients with no medicine. Retrieved from https://www.timesofisrael.com/medical-cannabis-reform-leaves-at-least-5000-patients-with-no-medicine/. (Accessed 7 September 2020.)

Lu, M.L., & Agito, M.D. (2015). Cannabinoid hyperemesis syndrome: Marijuana is both antiemetic and proemetic. *Cleveland Clinic Journal of Medicine*, 82(7), 429–434.

Main Department of Administrative and Financial Services. (2020). Maine medical use of marijuana program: January 1, 2019–December 31, 2019 annual report to the Maine State Legislature. Retrieved from https://www.maine.gov/dafs/omp/sites/maine.gov.dafs.omp/files/inline-files/office-of-marijuana-policy_dafs_mmmp-annual-report-2019.pdf . (Accessed 7 September 2020.)

Medical Cannabis Network. (2020). Medical cannabis prescriptions: three years of cannabis law in Germany. Retrieved from https://www.healtheuropa. eu/medical-cannabis-prescriptions-three-years-of-cannabis-law-in-germany/97628/. (Accessed 7 September 2020.)

National Academies of Sciences, Engineering, and Medicine. (2017). The health effects of cannabis and cannabinoids: The current state of the evidence and recommendations for research. Washington, DC: The National Academies Press.

National Conference of State Legislatures. (2019). Marijuana overview. Retrieved from https://www.ncsl.org/research/civil-and-criminal-justice/ marijuana-overview.aspx. (Accessed 7 September 2020.)

National Conference of State Legislatures. (2020). State medical marijuana laws. Retrieved from https://www.ncsl.org/research/health/state-medical-marijuana-laws.aspx. (Accessed 7 September 2020.)

National Institutes of Health. (2020). Estimates of funding for various research, conditions, and disease categories (RCDC). Retrieved from https://report. nih.gov/categorical_spending.aspx. (Accessed 7 September 2020.)

Natural Medicines. (2020). Cannabis. Retrieved from https://naturalmedicines-therapeuticresearch-com.proxy.heal-wa.org/databases/food,-herbs-supplements/professional.aspx?productid=947. (Accessed 7 September 2020.)

New Hampshire Statutes. (2016). Title X – public health. Chapter 126-X – use of cannabis for therapeutic purposes. Retrieved from https://law.justia.com/ codes/new-hampshire/2016/title-x/chapter-126-x. (Accessed 7 September 2020.)

Osborn, L.A., Lauritsen, K.J., Cross, N., et al. (2015). Self-medication of somatic and psychiatric conditions using botanical marijuana. *Journal of Psychoactive Drugs*, 47(5), 345–350.

ProCon.org. (2018). Number of legal medical marijuana patients. Retrieved from https://medicalmarijuana.procon.org/number-of-legal-medical-marijuana-patients/. (Accessed 7 September 2020.)

ProCon.org. (2020). Legal medical marijuana states and DC: Laws, fees and possession limits. Retrieved from https://medicalmarijuana.procon.org/ legal-medical-marijuana-states-and-dc/. (Accessed 7 September 2020.)

Rosenthal, L.D., & Burchum, J.R. (2018). Lehne's pharmacotherapeutics for advanced practice providers. New York: Elsevier.

Russell, K., Cahill, M., Gowen, K., et al. (2018). The NCSBN national nursing guidelines for medical marijuana. *The Journal of Nursing Regulation*, 9(2), S1–S60.

Sessions, J.B. (2018). Marijuana enforcement. Retrieved from https://www.justice. gov/opa/press-release/file/1022196/download. (Accessed 7 September 2020.)

The American Legion. (2016). Resolution No. 11: Medical marijuana research. Retrieved from https://archive.legion.org/bitstream/handle/20.500.12203/ 5763/2016n011.pdf?sequence=4&isallowed=y. (Accessed 7 September 2020.)

UNIMED Pharmaceuticals. (2004). Marinol® (dronabinol) capsules. Retrieved from https://www.accessdata.fda.gov/drugsatfda_docs/label/2005/018651s021lbl. pdf. (Accessed 7 September 2020.)

University of Michigan. (2018). National poll on healthy aging. Retrieved from https://deepblue.lib.umich.edu/bitstream/handle/2027.42/143211/ npha%20marijuana%20report.pdf?sequence=1&isallowed=y.

US Food and Drug Administration. (2020a). FDA and cannabis: Research and drug approval process. Retrieved from https://www.fda.gov/news-events/ public-health-focus/fda-and-cannabis-research-and-drug-approval-process. (Accessed 7 September 2020.)

US Food and Drug Administration. (2020b). FDA regulation of cannabis and cannabis-derived products, including cannabidiol (CBD). Retrieved from https://www.fda.gov/news-events/public-health-focus/fda-regulation-cannabis-and-cannabis-derived-products-including-cannabidiol-cbd#whatare. (Accessed 7 September 2020.)

Valeant Pharmaceuticals International. (2006). Cesamet™ (nabilone) capsules. Retrieved from https://www.accessdata.fda.gov/drugsatfda_docs/label/ 2006/018677s011lbl.pdf. (Accessed 7 September 2020.)

Vermont Department of Public Safety. (2020). Marijuana registry: Medical and mental health professionals. Retrieved from https://medicalmarijuana.vermont. gov/medical-and-mental-health-professionals. (Accessed 7 September 2020.)

Washington State Legislature. (2019). Medical cannabis: Crimes – limitations of chapter. RCW 69.51A.060 (2). Retrieved from https://app.leg.wa.gov/rcw/ default.aspx?cite=69.51A.060. (Accessed 7 September 2020.)

Wikipedia. (2020). Legality of cannabis. Retrieved from https://en.wikipedia. org/wiki/Legality_of_cannabis. (Accessed 7 September 2020.)

Wilsey, B., Atkinson, J.H., Marcotte, T.D., & Grant, I. (2015). The medicinal cannabis treatment agreement: providing information to chronic pain patients via a written document. *Clinical Journal of Pain*, 31(12), 1087–1096.

Index

The Advanced Practice Registered Nurse as a Prescriber, Second Edition. Edited by Louise Kaplan and Marie Annette Brown.
© 2021 John Wiley & Sons Ltd. Published 2021 by John Wiley & Sons Ltd.